T0348619

Regional Anesthesia

Editors

NABIL M. ELKASSABANY
EDWARD R. MARIANO

ANESTHESIOLOGY CLINICS

www.anesthesiology.theclinics.com

Consulting Editor
LEE A. FLEISHER

September 2018 • Volume 36 • Number 3

ELSEVIER

1600 John F. Kennedy Boulevard • Suite 1800 • Philadelphia, Pennsylvania, 19103-2899

http://www.theclinics.com

ANESTHESIOLOGY CLINICS Volume 36, Number 3
September 2018 ISSN 1932-2275, ISBN-13: 978-0-323-61372-9

Editor: Colleen Dietzler
Developmental Editor: Kristen Helm

Anesthesiology Clinics (ISSN 1932-2275) is published quarterly by Elsevier Inc., 360 Park Avenue South, New York, NY 10010-1710. Months of issue are March, June, September, and December. Periodicals postage paid at New York, NY and at additional mailing offices. Subscription prices are $100.00 per year (US student/resident), $346.00 per year (US individuals), $437.00 per year (Canadian individuals), $657.00 per year (US institutions), $830.00 per year (Canadian institutions), $225.00 per year (Canadian and foreign student/resident), $460.00 per year (foreign individuals), and $830.00 per year (foreign institutions). To receive student and resident rate, orders must be accompanied by name of affiliated institution, date of term, and the *signature* of program/residency coordinator on institutions letterhead. Orders will be billed at individual rate until proof of status is received. Foreign air speed delivery is included in all *Clinics'* subscription prices. All prices are subject to change without notice. POSTMASTER: Send address changes to *Anesthesiology Clinics,* Elsevier Health Sciences Division, Subscription Customer Service, 3251 Riverport Lane, Maryland Heights, MO 63043. Customer Service (orders, claims, online, change of address): Elsevier Health Sciences Division, Subscription Customer Service, 3251 Riverport Lane, Maryland Heights, MO 63043. **Tel:1-800-654-2452 (U.S. and Canada); 314-447-8871 (outside U.S. and Canada). Fax: 314-447-8029. E-mail: journalscustomerservice-usa@elsevier. com (for print support); journalsonlinesupport-usa@elsevier.com (for online support).**

Reprints. For copies of 100 or more of articles in this publication, please contact the Commercial Reprints Department Elsevier Inc., 360 Park Avenue South, New York, NY 10010-1710. Tel.: 212-633-3874; Fax: 212-633-3820; E-mail reprints@elsevier.com.

Anesthesiology Clinics, is also published in Spanish by McGraw-Hill Inter-americana Editores S. A., P.O. Box 5-237 06500 Mexico D. F., Mexico.

Anesthesiology Clinics, is covered in *MEDLINE/PubMed (Index Medicus), Current Contents/Clinical Medicine, Excerpta Medica, ISI/BIOMED,* and *Chemical Abstracts.*

Contributors

CONSULTING EDITOR

LEE A. FLEISHER, MD
Robert D. Dripps Professor and Chair of Anesthesiology and Critical Care, Professor of Medicine, Perelman School of Medicine, University of Pennsylvania, Philadelphia, Pennsylvania, USA

EDITORS

NABIL M. ELKASSABANY, MD, MSCE
Director, Sections of Orthopedic and Regional Anesthesiology, Associate Professor, Department of Anesthesiology and Critical Care, Perelman School of Medicine, University of Pennsylvania, Philadelphia, Pennsylvania, USA

EDWARD R. MARIANO, MD, MAS (Clinical Research)
Chief, Anesthesiology and Perioperative Care Service, Associate Chief of Staff for Inpatient Surgical Services, VA Palo Alto Health Care System, Professor of Anesthesiology, Perioperative and Pain Medicine, Stanford School of Medicine, Palo Alto, California, USA

AUTHORS

ANUJ KAILASH AGGARWAL, MD
Pain Medicine Fellow, Department of Anesthesiology, Perioperative and Pain Medicine, Stanford School of Medicine, Redwood City, California, USA

SIBLE ANTONY, MD
Fellow in Pediatric Anesthesiology, Department of Anesthesiology and Critical Care, The Children's Hospital of Philadelphia, Philadelphia, Pennsylvania, USA

JAIME L. BARATTA, MD
Clinical Assistant Professor, Department of Anesthesiology, Sidney Kimmel Medical College, Thomas Jefferson University, Philadelphia, Pennsylvania, USA

VALENTINA BELLINI, MD
Department of Anesthesia and Pain Therapy, Parma University Hospital, Parma, Italy

DARIO BUGADA, MD
SIMPAR Group (Study in Multidisciplinary Pain Research), Emergency and Intensive Care Department, ASST Papa Giovanni XXIII, Bergamo, Italy

AMIR C. DAYAN, MD
Clinical Instructor, Department of Anesthesiology, Sidney Kimmel Medical College, Thomas Jefferson University, Philadelphia, Pennsylvania, USA

NABIL M. ELKASSABANY, MD, MSCE
Director, Sections of Orthopedic and Regional Anesthesiology, Associate Professor, Department of Anesthesiology and Critical Care, Perelman School of Medicine, University of Pennsylvania, Philadelphia, Pennsylvania, USA

RODNEY A. GABRIEL, MD, MAS (Clinical Research)
Assistant Clinical Professor, Department of Anesthesiology, University of California, San Diego, San Diego, California, USA

JEFF GADSDEN, MD, FRCPC, FANZCA
Associate Professor, Department of Anesthesiology, Duke University Medical Center, Durham, North Carolina, USA

ARJUNAN GANESH, MBBS
Associate Professor of Anesthesiology, Department of Anesthesiology and Critical Care, The Children's Hospital of Philadelphia, Perelman School of Medicine, University of Pennsylvania, Philadelphia, Pennsylvania, USA

STUART A. GRANT, MB ChB
Professor, Department of Anesthesiology, Duke University Medical Center, Durham, North Carolina, USA

TARAS GROSH, MD
Assistant Professor, Department of Anesthesiology and Critical Care, Perelman School of Medicine, University of Pennsylvania, Philadelphia, Pennsylvania, USA

HARSHAD GURNANEY, MBBS, MPH
Associate Professor of Anesthesiology, Department of Anesthesiology and Critical Care, The Children's Hospital of Philadelphia, Perelman School of Medicine, University of Pennsylvania, Philadelphia, Pennsylvania, USA

THOMAS KYLE HARRISON, MD
Clinical Associate Professor (Affiliated), Department of Anesthesiology, Perioperative and Pain Medicine, Stanford School of Medicine, Staff Physician, VA Palo Alto Health Care System, Palo Alto, California, USA

BRIAN M. ILFELD, MD, MS (Clinical Investigation)
Professor (in residence), Department of Anesthesiology, University of California, San Diego, San Diego, California, USA

T. EDWARD KIM, MD
Director of Regional Anesthesia and Acute Pain Medicine, Anesthesiology and Perioperative Care Service, VA Palo Alto Health Care System, Palo Alto, California, USA; Associate Clinical Professor (affiliated), Department of Anesthesiology, Perioperative and Pain Medicine, Stanford School of Medicine, Stanford, California, USA

HOWARD KORNFELD, MD
Clinical Faculty, Pain Fellowship Program, University of California, San Francisco School of Medicine, Mill Valley, California, USA

AMANDA H. KUMAR, MD
Assistant Professor, Department of Anesthesiology, Duke University Medical Center, Durham, North Carolina, USA

LISA KUMAR, MD
Fellow, Regional Anesthesiology and Acute Pain Medicine, Department of Anesthesiology, Duke University Medical Center, Durham, North Carolina, USA

ANNA LEMBKE, MD
Associate Professor, Departments of Psychiatry and Behavioral Sciences, and Anesthesiology and Pain Medicine, Stanford School of Medicine, Stanford, California, USA

LUCA F. LORINI, MD
Chairman, Emergency and Intensive Care Department, ASST Papa Giovanni XXIII, Bergamo, Italy

EDWARD R. MARIANO, MD, MAS (Clinical Research)
Chief, Anesthesiology and Perioperative Care Service, Associate Chief of Staff for Inpatient Surgical Services, VA Palo Alto Health Care System, Professor of Anesthesiology, Perioperative and Pain Medicine, Stanford School of Medicine, Palo Alto, California, USA

STAVROS G. MEMTSOUDIS, MD, PhD, FCCP
Clinical Professor of Anesthesiology and Public Health, Department of Anesthesiology, Weill Cornell Medical College, Senior Scientist, Attending Anesthesiologist, Hospital for Special Surgery, New York, New York, USA

DARSI N. PITCHON, MD
Clinical Instructor, Department of Anesthesiology, Sidney Kimmel Medical College, Thomas Jefferson University, Philadelphia, Pennsylvania, USA

RON E. SAMET, MD
Assistant Professor, Department of Anesthesiology, Division of Trauma Anesthesiology, R Adams Cowley Shock Trauma Center, University of Maryland Medical Center, University of Maryland School of Medicine, Baltimore, Maryland, USA

ERIC S. SCHWENK, MD, FASA
Associate Professor, Department of Anesthesiology, Sidney Kimmel Medical College, Thomas Jefferson University, Philadelphia, Pennsylvania, USA

IAN R. SLADE, MD
Assistant Professor, Department of Anesthesiology and Pain Medicine, Harborview Medical Center, University of Washington School of Medicine, Seattle, Washington, USA

EUGENE R. VISCUSI, MD
Professor, Department of Anesthesiology, Sidney Kimmel Medical College, Thomas Jefferson University, Philadelphia, Pennsylvania, USA

CHRISTOPHER A.J. WEBB, MD
Director of Regional Anesthesiology and Acute Pain Medicine, Department of Anesthesiology and Perioperative Medicine, Kaiser Permanente South San Francisco Medical Center, Adjunct Assistant Clinical Professor, Department of Anesthesia and Perioperative Care, University of California, San Francisco School of Medicine, San Francisco, California, USA

Contents

Foreword: Regional Anesthesia: What We Need to Know in the Era of
Enhanced Recovery After Surgery Protocols and the Opioid Epidemic   xi

Lee A. Fleisher

Preface: Regional Anesthesiology and Acute Pain Medicine in the Era of
Value-Based Health Care   xiii

Nabil M. Elkassabany and Edward R. Mariano

Establishing an Acute Pain Service in Private Practice and Updates on
Regional Anesthesia Billing   333

Christopher A.J. Webb and T. Edward Kim

Acute pain management is an expanding perioperative specialty, and there is a renewed focus on implementing and developing an acute pain service (APS) in nonacademic hospitals (ie, "private practice"). An anesthesiologist-led APS can improve patient care by decreasing perioperative morbidity and potentially reducing the risk of chronic postsurgical pain syndromes. Elements of a successful APS include multidisciplinary collaboration to develop perioperative pain protocols, education of health care providers and patients, and regular evaluation of patient safety and quality-of-care metrics. Standardization of regional anesthesia procedures and billing practices can promote consistent outcomes and efficiency.

Perioperative Considerations for the Patient with Opioid Use Disorder on
Buprenorphine, Methadone, or Naltrexone Maintenance Therapy   345

Thomas Kyle Harrison, Howard Kornfeld, Anuj Kailash Aggarwal,
and Anna Lembke

As part of a national effort to combat the current US opioid epidemic, use of currently Food and Drug Administration–approved drugs for the treatment of opioid use disorder/opioid addiction (buprenorphine, methadone, and naltrexone) is on the rise. To provide optimal pain control and minimize the risk of relapse and overdose, providers need to have an in-depth understanding of how to manage these medications in the perioperative setting. This article reviews key principles and discusses perioperative considerations for patients with opioid use disorder on buprenorphine, methadone, or naltrexone.

Updates on Multimodal Analgesia for Orthopedic Surgery   361

Darsi N. Pitchon, Amir C. Dayan, Eric S. Schwenk, Jaime L. Baratta,
and Eugene R. Viscusi

Pain control after orthopedic surgery is challenging. A multimodal approach provides superior analgesia with fewer side effects compared with opioids alone. This approach is particularly useful in light of the current opioid epidemic in the United States. Several new nonopioid agents have emerged into the market in recent years. New agents included in this article are intravenous acetaminophen, intranasal ketorolac, and newer nonsteroidal antiinflammatory drugs and the established medications ketamine and gabapentinoids. This article evaluates the evidence supporting these drugs in a multimodal context, including a brief discussion of cost.

Updates in Enhanced Recovery Pathways for Total Knee Arthroplasty   375

Lisa Kumar, Amanda H. Kumar, Stuart A. Grant, and Jeff Gadsden

Enhanced recovery after surgery (ERAS) programs for orthopedics involve a multidisciplinary approach to accelerating return to function, reducing pain, improving patient comfort and satisfaction, reducing complications from the surgical procedure, reducing hospital length of stay, and reducing costs. ERAS pathways for patients receiving total knee arthroplasty are different from those having intracavitary surgery; they are less focused on fluid homeostasis and gut motility than they are on optimizing systemic and local analgesics and providing a balance between the highest-quality pain control and accelerated return to ambulation.

Novel Methodologies in Regional Anesthesia for Knee Arthroplasty   387

Rodney A. Gabriel and Brian M. Ilfeld

Maximizing analgesia is critical following joint arthroplasty because postoperative pain is a major barrier to adequate physical therapy. Continuous peripheral nerve blocks have been the mainstay for acute pain management in this population; however, this and similar techniques are limited by their duration of action. Cryoneurolysis and peripheral nerve stimulation are two methodologies used for decades to treat chronic pain. With the advent of portable ultrasound devices and percutaneous administration equipment, both procedures may now be suitable for the treatment of acute pain. This article reviews these two modalities and their application to joint arthroplasty.

Update on Selective Regional Analgesia for Hip Surgery Patients   403

Dario Bugada, Valentina Bellini, Luca F. Lorini, and Edward R. Mariano

In hip surgery, regional anesthesia offers benefits in pain management and recovery. There are a wide range of regional analgesic options; none have been shown to be superior. Lumbar plexus block, femoral nerve block, and fascia iliaca block are the most supported by the published literature. Other techniques, such as selective obturator and/or lateral femoral cutaneous nerve blocks, represent alternatives. Newer approaches, such as quadratus lumborum block and local infiltration analgesia, require rigorous studies. To realize long-term outcome benefits, postoperative regional analgesia must be tailored to the individual patient and last longer.

Enhanced Recovery After Shoulder Arthroplasty   417

Taras Grosh and Nabil M. Elkassabany

Enhanced recovery after surgery (ERAS) protocols depend on multidisciplinary care and should be peer reviewed and data driven. ERAS has reduced hospital length of stay and complications, simultaneously improving patient outcomes. The ERAS protocol after shoulder arthroplasty features multidisciplinary collaboration among different perioperative services and multimodal analgesia, with a focus on regional anesthesia. Despite success of this protocol, adoption is not universal because ERAS protocols are resource intensive. They require clinicians invested in the success of these programs and patients who can take charge of their own health. Future protocols need to include quality-of-life and functional outcome measures to gauge success from the patient perspective.

Regional Anesthesia and Analgesia for Acute Trauma Patients   431

Ian R. Slade and Ron E. Samet

Regional anesthesia for the acute trauma patient is increasing because of the growing appreciation of its benefits, development of newer techniques and equipment, and more robust training. Block procedures are expanding beyond perioperative interventions performed exclusively by anesthesiologists to paramedics on scene, emergency medicine physicians, and nurse-led services using these techniques early in trauma pain management. Special considerations and indications apply to survivors of trauma compared with the elective patient and must be appreciated to optimize safety and clinical outcomes. This article discusses the current literature and future directions in the growing role of regional anesthesia in acute trauma care.

Pediatric Ambulatory Continuous Peripheral Nerve Blocks   455

Bible Antony, Harshad Gurnaney, and Arjunan Ganesh

Despite the widespread use of ambulatory continuous peripheral nerve blocks in adults, their use in children has been sporadic. Indications for the use of ambulatory continuous peripheral nerve block in children involve orthopedic procedure, whereby significant pain is anticipated beyond 24 hours. Techniques to place the perineural catheters in children are similar to that used in adults. The incidence of serious side effects in pediatric ambulatory continuous peripheral nerve block is extremely rare. When this is combined with the potential to increase patient and family satisfaction and decrease opioid-related side effects, ambulatory continuous peripheral nerve block becomes a compelling choice.

What Can Regional Anesthesiology and Acute Pain Medicine Learn from
"Big Data"?   467

Nabil M. Elkassabany, Stavros G. Memtsoudis, and Edward R. Mariano

Demonstrating value added to patients' experience through regional anesthesiology and acute pain medicine is critical. Evidence supporting improved outcomes can be derived from prospective studies or retrospective cohort studies. Population-based studies relying on existing clinical and administrative databases are helpful when an outcome is rare, and detecting a change would require studying large numbers of patients. This article discusses the effect of regional anesthesiology and acute pain medicine interventions on mortality and morbidity, infection rate, cancer recurrence, inpatient falls, local anesthetic systemic toxicity, persistent postsurgical pain, and health care costs.

ANESTHESIOLOGY CLINICS

FORTHCOMING ISSUES

December 2018
Preoperative Evaluation
Zdravka Zafirova and Richard D. Urman, *Editors*

March 2019
Cutting-Edge Trauma and Emergency Care
Maureen McCunn, Mohammed Iqbal Ahmed, and Catherine M. Kuza, *Editors*

June 2019
Ambulatory Anesthesia
Michael T. Walsh, *Editor*

RECENT ISSUES

June 2018
Practice Management: Successfully Guiding Your Group into the Future
Amr E. Abouleish and Stanley W. Stead, *Editors*

March 2018
Quality Improvement and Implementation Science
Meghan B. Lane-Fall and Lee A. Fleisher, *Editors*

December 2017
Anesthesia Outside the Operating Room
Mark S. Weiss and Wendy L. Gross, *Editors*

RELATED INTEREST

Orthopedic Clinics of North America, October 2017 (Vol. 48, No. 4)
Perioperative Pain Management
Clayton C. Bettin, James H. Calandruccio, Benjamin J. Grear, Benjamin M. Mauck, Jeffrey R. Sawyer, Patrick C. Toy, and John C. Weinlein, *Editors*
Available at: http://www.orthopedic.theclinics.com/

THE CLINICS ARE AVAILABLE ONLINE!
Access your subscription at:
www.theclinics.com

Foreword

Regional Anesthesia: What We Need to Know in the Era of Enhanced Recovery After Surgery Protocols and the Opioid Epidemic

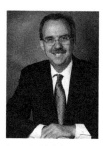

Lee A. Fleisher, MD
Consulting Editor

Over the past decade, there has become increasing evidence on the negative effects of opioids as a primary modality for perioperative pain management. Enhanced Recovery after Surgery (ERAS) has become a standard approach to surgical care in many hospitals as a means of reducing length of stay with similar or improved outcomes compared to traditional strategies. Multimodal analgesia is a mainstay of ERAS, and regional anesthesia offers the ability to both reduce the need for general anesthetics and improve postoperative pain management and return to both physical and bowel function. In addition, postoperative opioid-prescribing techniques have contributed to the opioid epidemic in the United States, and opioid-sparing techniques, which could include regional anesthesia, can help reduce the needs for postoperative narcotics. This issue of *Anesthesiology Clinics* can provide insights into both areas.

This issue was proposed by two leaders in thought in this arena, Nabil M. Elkassabany, MD, MSCE and Edward R. Mariano, MD, MAS (Clinical Research). Dr Elkassabany is Associate Professor of Anesthesiology and Critical Care at the Hospital of the University of Pennsylvania. He is the director of the section of Orthopedic and Regional Anesthesiology. Dr Mariano is Professor of Anesthesiology, Perioperative and Pain Medicine with a Master of Advanced Studies Degree in Clinical Research. He serves as Chief of the Anesthesiology and Perioperative Care Service and Associate Chief of Staff for Inpatient Surgical Services at the Veterans Affairs Palo Alto Health Care System and Program Director of the Stanford Regional Anesthesiology and Acute Pain Medicine Fellowship Program. They are both on the Board of Directors

Anesthesiology Clin 36 (2018) xi–xii
https://doi.org/10.1016/j.anclin.2018.06.002
1932-2275/18/© 2018 Published by Elsevier Inc.

of the American Society of Regional Anesthesia and Pain Management. Together, they have created a provocative and timely issue of the *Anesthesiology Clinics*.

Lee A. Fleisher, MD
Perelman School of Medicine at
University of Pennsylvania
3400 Spruce Street, Dulles 680
Philadelphia, PA 19104, USA

E-mail address:
Lee.Fleisher@uphs.upenn.edu

Preface

Regional Anesthesiology and Acute Pain Medicine in the Era of Value-Based Health Care

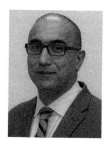
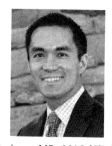

Nabil M. Elkassabany, MD, MSCE   Edward R. Mariano, MD, MAS (Clinical Research)
Editors

The practice of regional anesthesia has gone through a noticeable transformation. Now defined by the Accreditation Council for Graduate Medical Education (ACGME) as a subspecialty of anesthesiology, developments in regional anesthesiology and acute pain medicine offer effective alternatives to general anesthesia and form the basis of opioid-sparing multimodal analgesia for surgical patients. For the past 50 years, study after study has examined the quality of postoperative pain management resulting from peripheral nerve and neuraxial blockade, yet the results consistently show that most patients still complain of significant pain after surgery. We still have work to do.

Throughout the history of regional anesthesia research, a primary focus has been the technical aspects of performing procedures—whether needle placement in location X versus location Y will result in better blocks. While expertise in relevant anatomy, pharmacology, and needle skills are *necessary* elements for successful implementation of regional anesthesiology and acute pain medicine, these elements are not *sufficient*. The goals of today's regional anesthesiology and acute pain medicine specialists have gone way beyond the "block." They now have embraced the role of physician leaders and are poised to disseminate and implement new perioperative care models.

This issue of *Anesthesiology Clinics* is a reflection of this viewpoint. We are grateful to the series editor, Dr Fleisher, for the opportunity to present a collection of articles that reflect the evolution of regional anesthesiology and acute pain medicine. This editorial collaboration is an exciting new project for the two of us. For the past several years, we have worked together on many projects promoting the subspecialty of regional anesthesiology and acute pain medicine: developing the competency-based milestones for the newly ACGME-accredited regional anesthesiology and acute pain medicine fellowships; working together on the American Society of Regional

Anesthesiology Clin 36 (2018) xiii–xiv
https://doi.org/10.1016/j.anclin.2018.06.001
1932-2275/18/© 2018 Published by Elsevier Inc.

anesthesiology.theclinics.com

Anesthesia and Pain Medicine (ASRA) communications committees and ASRA Board of Directors; developing national quality measures in pain management; collaborating on clinical research projects; and coediting a previous issue of *Anesthesiology Clinics* on "Orthopedic Anesthesiology." In this issue, we have carefully selected articles that highlight the value that regional anesthesia offers patients and how physicians can establish their own programs in regional anesthesiology and acute pain medicine in various practice settings. These topics include building an ambulatory perineural catheter program for pediatric patients, the use of regional anesthesia in trauma patients, and establishing enhanced recovery protocols for joint arthroplasty patients. We also cover some timely and challenging topics: managing patients on opioid replacement therapy, newer drugs on the horizon for multimodal analgesia, new frontiers and technologies in regional anesthesia, and the use of "big data" to study the most important outcomes that matter to our patients.

We are grateful for our families for their unwavering support, our authors for donating their time and expertise, and the readership of *Anesthesiology Clinics*. It is our hope that this final product represents an up-to-date comprehensive review of the most pressing issues pertaining to value-based regional anesthesiology and acute pain medicine and offers something for everyone.

Nabil M. Elkassabany, MD, MSCE
Sections of Orthopedic and Regional Anesthesiology
Department of Anesthesiology and Critical Care
Perelman School of Medicine
University of Pennsylvania
3400 Spruce Street, Dulles 7th
Philadelphia, PA 19104, USA

Edward R. Mariano, MD, MAS (Clinical Research)
Department of Anesthesiology
Perioperative and Pain Medicine
Stanford University School of Medicine
Anesthesiology and Perioperative Care Service
VA Palo Alto Health Care System
3801 Miranda Avenue (112A)
Palo Alto, CA 94304, USA

E-mail addresses:
Nabil.Elkassabany@uphs.upenn.edu (N.M. Elkassabany)
emariano@stanford.edu (E.R. Mariano)

Establishing an Acute Pain Service in Private Practice and Updates on Regional Anesthesia Billing

Christopher A.J. Webb, MD[a,b], T. Edward Kim, MD[c,d],*

KEYWORDS

- Acute pain service • Postoperative pain • Private practice • Regional anesthesia
- Billing

KEY POINTS

- Pain management by an acute pain service (APS) can improve patient outcomes such as decreasing pain intensity, increasing patient satisfaction, shortening hospital length of stay, and decreasing risk of persistent postsurgical pain syndrome.
- An APS can implement and sustain perioperative pain management protocols that include regional anesthesia for postsurgical patients.
- Roles of an APS include individualized postoperative pain management, education of health care providers, assessment of patient safety and quality of care, and institution of established billing practices.
- A successful APS will require multidisciplinary collaboration as well as support from members of the anesthesiology group.
- When establishing a peripheral nerve block program, it is recommended to focus on 1 or 2 surgical patient populations and then gradually expand to other surgical specialties.

Financial Support: None.

Disclosure Statement: The authors have nothing to disclose.

[a] Department of Anesthesiology and Perioperative Medicine, Kaiser Permanente South San Francisco Medical Center, 1200 El Camino Real, South San Francisco, CA 94080, USA; [b] Department of Anesthesia and Perioperative Care, University of California San Francisco School of Medicine, 521 Parnassus Avenue, San Francisco, CA 94143, USA; [c] Anesthesiology and Perioperative Care Service, Veterans Affairs Palo Alto Health Care System, 3801 Miranda Avenue (112A), Palo Alto, CA 94304, USA; [d] Department of Anesthesiology, Perioperative and Pain Medicine, Stanford University School of Medicine, 300 Pasteur Drive, Stanford, CA 94305, USA

* Corresponding author. Anesthesiology and Perioperative Care Service. VA Palo Health Care System, 3801 Miranda Avenue (112A), Palo Alto, CA 94304.

E-mail address: tekim@stanford.edu

Anesthesiology Clin 36 (2018) 333–344

https://doi.org/10.1016/j.anclin.2018.04.005

1932-2275/18/Published by Elsevier Inc.

anesthesiology.theclinics.com

INTRODUCTION

Postoperative pain management is one of the primary concerns for patients undergoing surgery[1,2] and a cause of delayed hospital discharge.[3] Benefits of adequate postoperative pain control include decreased patient morbidity[4–6] and mortality[7] and potential reduction of persistent postsurgical[8,9] and chronic[10] pain. Although many opioid and nonopioid analgesic modalities currently exist for treatment of pain, it is recommended that such treatments occur within the context of an organized acute pain service (APS)[11] with additional emphasis on physicians with subspecialty training in acute pain medicine.[12] Implementation of an APS at nonacademic hospitals is not only feasible but necessary to ensure that patients are offered the highest quality of acute pain management.

ROLES AND RESPONSIBILITIES OF AN ACUTE PAIN SERVICE

Since the initial descriptions of an APS,[13,14] hospitals worldwide have initiated analogous services for treating acute postoperative pain.[2,15–18] Although the roles of an APS have evolved over the years, the current practice of acute pain medicine involves assessment, treatment, and management of acute pain using multimodal analgesia[11] that may include interventional procedures. Regional anesthesia and acute pain medicine (RAAPM) is a rapidly developing subspecialty of anesthesiology, and anesthesiologists who are trained or have expertise in RAAPM are uniquely positioned to be leaders in their hospitals to develop, implement, and direct acute pain services.[12] Although the daily activities of an APS can differ depending on the practice setting, the general responsibilities of an APS typically involve consistent clinical practice of evidenced-based care, education of health care providers and patients, generation of revenue by instituting established billing practices, and performance of routine audits to assess quality of care and patient safety.

Patient Care

One of the most important roles of an APS is to develop surgery-specific pain management protocols and enhanced recovery pathways. Clinical pathways delineate sequence and timing of evidenced-based interventions and coordinate activities of physicians, nurses, and other health care providers.[14] Multimodal analgesic therapies are recommended[11] and can be integrated into clinical pathways. However, studies in Europe and United States have shown that postoperative pain management protocols are not commonplace[15,16] and utilization of multimodal analgesic therapies can vary dramatically depending on local hospital culture and physician preferences.[17] The added value of an APS is having dedicated specialists implement and sustain protocols or clinical pathways through daily care of surgical patients during the perioperative period. Having an APS was shown to be critical in adherence to an interdisciplinary clinical pathway for surgery[18] and is associated with statistically significant decrease in postoperative pain scores.[19]

The primary clinical responsibility of an APS is to perform daily assessments of acute pain patients and provide individualized treatment plans. This can include management of neuraxial or peripheral nerve block (PNB) procedures for hospitalized patients as well as making "telephone rounds" on patients at home with perineural catheter infusions. In regard to postoperative pain management, an APS can be available as a consultative service to assist "as needed," or arrangements can be made with surgeons to routinely manage patients with history of difficult postoperative pain control or patients at risk for chronic opioid use after surgery[20,21] and persistent postsurgical pain syndrome[22,23] (**Table 1**). An APS can also serve as a consultative

Table 1
Risk factors for persistent postsurgical pain

Preoperative	Intraoperative	Postoperative
Age < 40 y	Tissue ischemia	Uncontrolled acute pain
Female	Nerve damage	Sensory loss after surgery
Body mass index > 30 kg/m^2	Repeat surgery	Surgical complications (eg,
Preoperative pain (>1 mo)	Breast surgery	infection, hematoma, etc.)
History of chronic pain	Thoracotomy, coronary artery	Radiation therapy to surgical
Mood disorders (depression,	bypass surgery	site
anxiety, pain	Amputations	Neurotoxic medications (eg,
catastrophizing)	Inguinal hernia repair	chemotherapy)
Workers compensation	Cesarean section delivery	
Genetic		

Adapted from Tiippana E, Hamunen K, Heiskanen T, et al. New approach for treatment of prolonged postoperative pain: APS out-patient clinic. Scand J Pain 2016;12:21.

resource for acute pain management in nonsurgical patients in medicine wards, emergency departments, burn units, and hospice wards. To be successful, 24-h coverage is recommended,[13,16,24] including weekends and holidays, to address urgent issues and provide continuity of care. Patients treated by an APS report lower pain intensity scores; have less nausea, sedation, and pruritus; experience higher level of satisfaction; and have shorter hospital length of stay (LOS).[25]

Administrative Duties

Instituting and maintaining hospital policies is often a prerequisite for an APS, especially if new clinical practices or medications are introduced. The APS must work closely with surgeons, nurses, pharmacists, physical therapists, and hospital administrators to ensure that goals of patient care are aligned and patient safety concerns are addressed. Hospital policies should clearly delineate responsibilities of providers and standardize safe and reliable practices. The APS in conjunction with pharmacy staff need to identify which local anesthetics and other analgesic medications are on hospital formulary and select generally accepted regimens. Standardized medication order sets with specific concentrations have been shown to decrease prescribing errors.[26] In hospitals and ambulatory centers that use disposable PNB infusion devices, pharmacists should be regularly informed about anticipated surgical case volumes to ensure sufficient devices are available. Similarly, collaboration with facility logistics specialists (eg, medical equipment or supply chain administrators) is recommended to facilitate acquisition of commonly used equipment or supplies (eg, nerve block kits, needles, catheters).

Education of Patients and Providers

Education regarding postoperative pain can help improve patients' surgical experience and decrease health care costs.[26,27] Educating patients before the day of surgery on regional anesthesia techniques and/or anticipated postoperative pain protocols has been shown to decrease anxiety,[21] increase patient knowledge,[22] and improve patient satisfaction.[22,23] Patients who receive preoperative education on regional anesthesia techniques are more likely to receive regional anesthesia on the day of surgery[24]; however, the effects of education on postoperative pain levels have been variable.[21,25] For hospitals without a dedicated preoperative anesthesia clinic, education on postoperative pain management can potentially take place during the initial surgical consultation. Educational materials such as pamphlets or videos on regional anesthesia and pain medications can be shared with patients during these visits.

Education of nursing staff and other health care providers should be coordinated by the APS. During the initial implementation of pain management protocols, APS along with nurse educators or designated nursing "champions" should provide in-services about safe medication administration practices as well as potential side effects or adverse events. In addition, physical and occupational therapists should have a general understanding of what type of motor and sensory block is expected after patients receive regional anesthetic techniques. Periodic reevaluations and continuing education need to be provided to account for possible changes to staff (eg, turnover) and whenever policies are modified. Depending on the local anesthetic infusion device company, clinical representatives may be available to train nursing staff on how to connect infusion devices to indwelling perineural catheters using sterile techniques, initiate a basal infusion, safely remove catheters, and troubleshoot problems with infusion delivery systems.

Quality Assessment and Improvement

One of the ongoing efforts of an APS will be addressing issues related to quality of care and patient safety. Performing routine audits can identify whether clinical goals are being achieved[28,29] and present opportunities to collaborate with other providers to improve patient outcomes. For example, in a hospital where PNBs are performed for total knee and hip arthroplasty,hospital where PNBs are performed for total knee and hip arthroplasty, implementation of a multidisciplinary fall prevention program by an anesthesiologist-led APS can reduce rate of inpatient falls.[27] Other potential adverse events that should be monitored include medication side effects, neurologic complications, catheter-related infections, medication order errors, infusion device malfunctions, and patient complaints about inadequate pain control. When adverse events transpire, the APS can take the lead in identifying probable causes, formulating workable solutions, modifying policies, reinforcing patient and staff education, and effectuating practice or system changes.

IMPLEMENTATION OF AN ACUTE PAIN SERVICE

The initial steps in setting up an APS is identifying its members and creating a sustainable work flow. Depending on staffing resources at each facility, the construct of an APS will vary and the roles and responsibilities will likely change and expand over time. Throughout the existence of an APS, but especially during the initial implementation process, it is imperative that the APS collaborate closely with hospital administrators, surgeons, pharmacists, and nurses because the success of new protocols and pain treatments will require their support.

Organization

Depending on the size and staffing model of the anesthesiology group, either all or select members of the group will participate in APS duties. Ideally, an anesthesiologist with proficiency and experience in RAAPM will serve as the APS director who, if needed, can recruit 2 to 3 anesthesiologists to form a leadership team to assist with pain protocols, education of colleagues on PNBs, hospital staff in-servicing, and meetings with hospital administrators.

If hospital resources are available, the inclusion of acute pain advanced practice providers (eg, physician assistants, nurse practitioners, or clinical nurse specialists) can be a clinically and economically effective model.[30] Especially in settings in which anesthesiologists are assigned daily to operating room duties, advanced practice providers under the direction of the APS anesthesiologist can round on postoperative surgical patients, address patient and nursing issues, formulate appropriate analgesic regimens, respond to acute pain consults, and perform daily calls to patients at home with perineural catheter infusions. They can also assist with education of patients, caregivers, and staff as well as participate in policy changes and quality improvement projects. Advanced practice providers can also be considered to cover call overnight and/or during weekends.

If advanced practice providers are not an option, the anesthesiology group must rely on available staff. For example, the postcall anesthesiologist can perform inpatient rounds, communicate management changes to the nursing staff and surgical teams, and request follow-up from the anesthesiologist scheduler for the operating room. For groups with an active labor analgesia service, the management of acute pain patients can also be performed in part by the anesthesiologist assigned to cover labor and delivery. If the daily APS consists of a single anesthesiologist, collaboration with ward nurses should be considered.[31,32] Success with this model relies on education and training of selected ward nurses (eg, pain resource nurses or pain management champions) who will take the lead in teaching ward nurses how to execute postoperative pain treatment algorithms.[31] In-services on how to monitor and manage patient-controlled analgesia and epidural catheters as well as how to connect and troubleshoot PNB infusion devices will alleviate the workload of the on-call APS practitioner.

Regional Anesthesia

Depending on the staffing and scheduling model of the anesthesiology group, the APS may or may not function as a dedicated regional anesthesia team. For some private practice groups that use a physician-only model, assigning an anesthesiologist to perform perioperative regional anesthesia techniques without billing for other anesthesia services may be challenging and even financially impractical. For groups functioning within an anesthesia care model, having a dedicated APS regional anesthesia team that can work in parallel with concurrent cases has been shown to decrease anesthesia-controlled time and may allow for the addition of an extra case per day.[32]

During the nascent stages of a regional anesthesia program, it is recommended to focus on 1 or 2 surgical patient populations and then gradually expand to other surgical specialties. This approach will afford opportunities to assess outcomes, receive feedback, and make applicable systems changes to enhance the APS's efforts. If PNBs are being introduced into protocols for the first time, single-injection PNBs have the advantages of not requiring advanced training and additional equipment (eg, catheters and infusion devices) compared with performing continuous PNBs. However, continuous perineural infusion of local anesthetic is recommended for prolonged postoperative pain control[33] and is an evidence-based component of multimodal analgesic protocols for painful surgery.[34] For groups considering continuous PNBs, it is important to recognize the increased workload and cost in initiating and maintaining a successful perineural catheter program. A collaborative decision needs to be made about the type of infusion device to purchase balancing clinical features (eg, basal rate options, patient bolus feature, total fillable volume, etc.) and cost. Because both single-use (disposable) and reusable infusion pumps are commercially available, each group needs to assess how to best incorporate one or both types of devices for inpatients and outpatients. When a perineural catheter program is initiated, the APS should provide patients with specific information about expected sensory and motor block in the affected extremity, anticipated side effects (eg, leaking around insertion), indications to pause infusions, and removal of perineural catheters at home. Patients at home should also know how to contact the on-call APS when questions or urgent issues arise. For certain surgeries, physiotherapists will perform home visits, and in such scenarios, educating physical and occupational therapists on catheter site assessment as well as catheter removal will allow them to relay necessary information to the APS and assist patients with catheter removal. During initial discussions about continuous PNBs with surgeons, clinical considerations such as anticoagulation, weight-bearing status, and outpatient pain medication prescriptions need to be clarified and communicated to patients and other health care providers.

Billing and Coding for Regional Anesthesia

A complete review of billing practices is beyond the scope of this article. Subsequently, key points will be summarized and updates to a previously published billing article will be provided.[35] It is recommended that the APS meet with the hospital billing department, or billing company if applicable, to ensure compliance with established practices.

Generally, surgeons are reimbursed for postoperative pain management as part of a global surgical payment bundle. Regional anesthesia procedures performed by anesthesiologists for postoperative pain control, and not as part of the primary surgical anesthetic, can be billed separately if certain requirements are met. As per the National Correct Coding Initiative (NCCI) Policy Manual for Medicare Services,[36] epidurals and PNBs can be billed for postoperative pain management if surgeons request assistance with postoperative pain management, there is a procedure note in the patient's medical record, and the regional anesthetic technique is not the primary mode of intraoperative anesthesia (ie, if PNB will be reported for postoperative pain control, the primary surgical anesthetic must be "general anesthesia, subarachnoid injection, or epidural injection;" if the primary surgical anesthetic is "monitored anesthesia care, conscious sedation, or regional anesthesia by peripheral nerve block," PNB cannot be reported separately for postoperative pain management). If the APS will manage surgical patients for postoperative pain control after the end of the anesthesia service, the "surgeon is responsible to document in the medical record the reason care is being referred to the anesthesia practitioner.[36]"

Adopting systematic billing practices within the group can promote consistency and efficiency. A standardized procedure note can ensure proper reporting of procedural details and billing information. Components of a note can include name of referring physician; indication and site of procedure; description of technique (eg, asepsis, nerve localization modality like ultrasound guidance or nerve stimulation, etc.); local anesthetic name, concentration, and volume; complications, if any; and provider information (eg, name or identifier).[35] For billing, correct International Statistical Classification of Diseases and Related Health Problems (ICD) and Current Procedural Terminology (CPT) codes must be used. **Table 2** lists commonly used CPT codes for PNBs. For follow-up visits after day of surgery, CPT code 01996 is reported for management of epidural or subarachnoid drug administration.[36] For established inpatients with peripheral nerve catheters, evaluation and management codes 99231 to 99233 can be used depending on extent of patient interview and examination, complexity of decision-making, and time spent.[37] For acute pain consultations, codes 99251 to 99255 can be used based on similar criteria.[37]

If PNBs are performed for postoperative pain control, adding modifier -59 to CPT codes designates the procedure as a distinct and separate service and can help unbundle it from another service (ie, primary surgical anesthetic).[36] Subsets of modifier -59 were developed to provide reporting specificity and include XE (separate

Table 2
Current procedural terminology codes for peripheral nerve blocks

Type	Single Injection	Continuous Infusion
Abdominal plane[a] (TAP, rectus sheath)	64486 (unilateral) 64488 (bilateral)	64487 (unilateral) 64489 (bilateral)
Axillary	64417	—
Brachial plexus	64415	64416
Femoral	64447	64448
Ilioinguinal/iliohypogastric	64425	—
Intercostal	64420 (single nerve) 64421 (multiple nerves)	—
Lumbar plexus	—	64449
Other	64450	—
Paravertebral[a] (thoracic)	64461 (single site) 64462[b] (second and additional sites)	64463
Sciatic	64445	64446

Abbreviation: TAP, transversus abdominis plane.
[a] Indicates imaging is included when performed.
[b] Report separately in conjunction with 64461.
From American Medical Association. Current Procedural Terminology (CPT) 2018 Professional Edition. Chicago: American Medical Association; 2018; with permission.

encounter), XS (separate structure), XP (separate practitioner), and XU (unusual nonoverlapping service). Although these modifiers are not required per the 2018 NCCI policy manual, practitioners should become familiar with them because "NCCI will eventually require use of these modifiers rather than modifier 59....[36]" Other applicable modifiers for peripheral nerve block CPT codes include modifier -50 (bilateral procedures) and modifier -51 (multiple procedures on same extremity).[37]

If ultrasound guidance is used as the mode of nerve localization, a charge can be generated using CPT code 76942.[35] This code includes reimbursement for image acquisition and interpretation as well as maintenance and storage of ultrasound machines. If the ultrasound machine is not personally owned by the providing anesthesiologist, modifier -26 should be added to only bill for the professional fee. It should be noted that CPT codes for transversus abdominis plane blocks and paravertebral blocks already include imaging as part of the reimbursement (see **Table 2**); subsequently, providers should not report ultrasound use separately to avoid duplicate billing.

Potential Barriers and Implementation Strategies

One barrier for implementing an APS is cost.[38] Groups that are productivity based must factor the opportunity cost of managing acute pain patients instead of billing for surgical anesthesia services. One way to overcome this financial hurdle is hiring advanced practice providers who function under the direction of an anesthesiologist-led APS.[30,39,40] Because benefits of RAAPM include cost savings by decreasing LOS in hospital[41] and intensive care units,[42] as well as lowering patient morbidity[4–6] and mortality,[7] arguments can be made that hospitals can provide funds for advanced practice providers. Adequate pain management is a top priority for patients[43] and a main determinant of whether or not a patient recommends a hospital to others.[38] Although an APS may not generate substantial revenue for the hospital, the potential savings from decreased hospitalization costs in addition to potential growth in surgical volume from patients' recommendations may prove to be beneficial in the long run.

For an APS to be successful, it is imperative to have full support from members of the anesthesiology group. Furthermore, in certain models that will require APS participation of all group members, the service should be able to function regardless of which anesthesiologist is on call. Thus, a group must objectively assess its experience level in managing patients with complex pain as well as their ability to perform and manage PNBs. For practitioners needing additional PNB experience, attendance of a 1-day standardized course may help provide the skills necessary to place perineural catheters.[44] Simulation-based as well as self-directed study has been shown to improve ultrasound-guided regional anesthesia skills.[45] Because surgeons can be concerned about the unpredictable success rates of regional anesthesia techniques,[46] it is imperative that all members of the group obtain the training necessary to produce consistent and predictable block outcomes.

Surgeon "buy in" is essential to launching an APS program. Especially for an APS that will be involved with performing regional anesthesia, it is important to understand and address potential concerns of surgeons. A study demonstrated that although many surgeons recognize the benefits of regional anesthesia for postoperative pain control, the primary reasons for not favoring regional anesthesia are fear of case delays and unpredictable success rate.[46] Possible ways to improve efficiency and produce consistent outcomes include standardization of the group's techniques and supplies.[47] The group should decide in advance which PNBs will be performed and ideally use similar procedural techniques. In regard to nerve localization, studies have demonstrated that ultrasound guidance can result in faster sensory block onset time,[48] greater success in achieving surgical anesthesia,[49] and less time to place perineural catheters[50] compared with nerve stimulation alone. If ultrasound is adopted, further standardization of technique (ie, short- vs long-axis view, in-plane vs out-of-plane needle) can be considered by the group to produce consistent block effects and facilitate troubleshooting of perineural catheters. Similarly, having an algorithm for local anesthetic type (ie, short- vs long-acting), concentration, and volume will ensure predictable density of sensory blockade and duration. Time pressure was reported by nonacademic anesthesiologists to be a major obstacle in implementing a regional anesthesia program,[51] and a regional anesthesia induction area[47] (ie, "block room") located within the preoperative area or the postanesthesia care unit can minimize delays if procedures can be performed concurrently with surgical cases. A block room also allows for storage of and prompt access to block supplies, monitors, equipment, and emergency medications including treatment of local anesthetic systemic toxicity. For catheter placement, a block kit that includes sterile drapes and supplies should be considered to minimize preparation time.

FUTURE DIRECTION OF PERIOPERATIVE PAIN MEDICINE

The current state of opioid abuse in the United States[52,53] poses multiple challenges. Patients taking chronic opioids preoperatively are known to have higher postoperative opioid consumption, longer hospital LOS, increased rates of discharge to skilled nursing or rehabilitation facilities, and increased risk for perioperative respiratory depression.[54–56] Between 2002 and 2011, the incidence of in-hospital postoperative opioid overdose doubled in the United States and in-hospital mortality rate was 4 times greater for patients who overdosed compared with patients who did not.[57] Physician prescribing patterns of postoperative opioids, although well intended, can be oftentimes excessive[58–60] and may lead to chronic opioid use following major and minor surgery.[21,58] Similar to other comorbidities such as coronary artery disease or hypertension that warrant evaluation preoperatively, patients with chronic pain or patients at risk for postsurgical pain syndrome should undergo preoperative risk stratification and optimization. The idea of a transitional[22,61–63] or perioperative[64] pain service that can coordinate pain management before surgery and continue their care after patients are discharged from the hospital has gained interest to optimize perioperative pain and opioid use. The multidisciplinary makeup of such a team includes anesthesiologists trained in acute and/or chronic pain medicine, acute pain nurses, pain psychologists, physical therapists, and case managers.[63] The transitional or perioperative pain service can collaborate with APS to identify high-risk patients, taper preoperative opioids,[65] institute nonopioid analgesics, and develop a perioperative pain management plan.[61,63] By maximizing nonopioid analgesics, in addition to biofeedback and physical therapy, transitional services have been shown to reduce the amount of opioid used during the acute postoperative period[22] and may mitigate the progression to chronic postsurgical pain. Patients can also be referred early in their pain progression to chronic pain specialists who can further assist in the management of patients with complex pain.[22,62,63]

SUMMARY

Implementation of an APS can lead to improved patient outcomes. Keys to a successful APS include leadership by anesthesiologists, interdisciplinary coordination, education of patients and health care providers, standardization of regional anesthesia procedures, and systematic billing practices. Given the current focus on perioperative opioid use, an APS can provide individualized inpatient pain management, institute multimodal analgesia, and collaborate with other providers involved with perioperative pain management.

REFERENCES

1. Jenkins K, Grady D, Wong J, et al. Post-operative recovery: day surgery patients' preferences. Br J Anaesth 2001;86(2):272–4.

2. Warfield CA, Kahn CH. Acute pain management. Programs in U.S. hospitals and experiences and attitudes among U.S. adults. Anesthesiology 1995;83(5): 1090–4.

3. Pavlin DJ, Chen C, Penaloza DA, et al. Pain as a factor complicating recovery and discharge after ambulatory surgery. Anesth Analg 2002;95(3):627–34. Table of contents.

4. Ballantyne JC, Carr DB, deFerranti S, et al. The comparative effects of postoperative analgesic therapies on pulmonary outcome: cumulative meta-analyses of randomized, controlled trials. Anesth Analg 1998;86(3):598–612.

5. Beattie WS, Badner NH, Choi P. Epidural analgesia reduces postoperative myocardial infarction: a meta-analysis. Anesth Analg 2001;93(4):853–8.

6. Kehlet H, Holte K. Effect of postoperative analgesia on surgical outcome. Br J Anaesth 2001;87(1):62–72.

7. Rodgers A, Walker N, Schug S, et al. Reduction of postoperative mortality and morbidity with epidural or spinal anaesthesia: results from overview of randomised trials. BMJ 2000;321(7275):1493.

8. White PF, Kehlet H. Improving postoperative pain management: what are the unresolved issues? Anesthesiology 2010;112(1):220–5.

9. Joshi GP, Ogunnaike BO. Consequences of inadequate postoperative pain relief and chronic persistent postoperative pain. Anesthesiol Clin North America 2005; 23(1):21–36.

10. Chapman CR, Vierck CJ. The transition of acute postoperative pain to chronic pain: an integrative overview of research on mechanisms. J Pain 2017;18(4): 359.e1-38.

11. American Society of Anesthesiologists Task Force on Acute Pain Management. Practice guidelines for acute pain management in the perioperative setting: an updated report by the American Society of Anesthesiologists Task Force on Acute Pain Management. Anesthesiology 2012;116(2):248–73.

12. Tighe P, Buckenmaier CC 3rd, Boezaart AP, et al. Acute pain medicine in the United States: a status report. Pain Med 2015;16(9):1806–26.

13. Ready LB, Oden R, Chadwick HS, et al. Development of an anesthesiology-based postoperative pain management service. Anesthesiology 1988;68(1): 100–6.

14. Kim S, Losina E, Solomon DH, et al. Effectiveness of clinical pathways for total knee and total hip arthroplasty: literature review. J Arthroplasty 2003;18(1):69–74.

15. Benhamou D, Berti M, Brodner G, et al. Postoperative analgesic therapy observational survey (PATHOS): a practice pattern study in 7 central/southern European countries. Pain 2008;136(1–2):134–41.

16. Nasir D, Howard JE, Joshi GP, et al. A survey of acute pain service structure and function in United States hospitals. Pain Res Treat 2011;2011:934932.

17. Ladha KS, Patorno E, Huybrechts KF, et al. Variations in the use of perioperative multimodal analgesic therapy. Anesthesiology 2016;124(4):837–45.

18. Steckelberg RC, Funck N, Kim TE, et al. Adherence to a multimodal analgesic clinical pathway: a within-group comparison of staged bilateral knee arthroplasty patients. Reg Anesth Pain Med 2017;42(3):368–71.

19. Werner MU, Soholm L, Rotboll-Nielsen P, et al. Does an acute pain service improve postoperative outcome? Anesth Analg 2002;95(5):1361–72. Table of contents.

20. Sun EC, Darnall BD, Baker LC, et al. Incidence of and risk factors for chronic opioid use among opioid-naive patients in the postoperative period. JAMA Intern Med 2016;176(9):1286–93.

21. Hah JM, Bateman BT, Ratliff J, et al. Chronic opioid use after surgery: implications for perioperative management in the face of the opioid epidemic. Anesth Analg 2017;125(5):1733–40.

22. Tiippana E, Hamunen K, Heiskanen T, et al. New approach for treatment of prolonged postoperative pain: APS out-patient clinic. Scand J Pain 2016;12:19–24.

23. Kehlet H, Jensen TS, Woolf CJ. Persistent postsurgical pain: risk factors and prevention. Lancet 2006;367(9522):1618–25.

24. Petrakis JK. Acute pain services in a community hospital. Clin J Pain 1989; 5(Suppl 1):S34–41.

25. Miaskowski C, Crews J, Ready LB, et al. Anesthesia-based pain services improve the quality of postoperative pain management. Pain 1999;80(1–2):23–9.

26. Louw A, Diener I, Landers MR, et al. Preoperative pain neuroscience education for lumbar radiculopathy: a multicenter randomized controlled trial with 1-year follow-up. Spine (Phila Pa 1976) 2014;39(18):1449–57.

27. Louw A, Diener I, Landers MR, et al. Three-year follow-up of a randomized controlled trial comparing preoperative neuroscience education for patients undergoing surgery for lumbar radiculopathy. J Spine Surg 2016;2(4):289–98.

28. Rawal N. Organization, function, and implementation of acute pain service. Anesthesiol Clin North America 2005;23(1):211–25.
29. Meissner W, Huygen F, Neugebauer EAM, et al. Management of acute pain in the postoperative setting: the importance of quality indicators. Curr Med Res Opin 2018;34(1):187–96.
30. Rawal N, Berggren L. Organization of acute pain services: a low-cost model. Pain 1994;57(1):117–23.
31. Gould TH, Crosby DL, Harmer M, et al. Policy for controlling pain after surgery: effect of sequential changes in management. BMJ 1992;305(6863):1187–93.
32. Chazapis M, Kaur N, Kamming D. Improving the peri-operative care of patients by instituting a 'block room' for regional anaesthesia. BMJ Qual Improv Rep 2014;3(1) [pii:u204061.w1769].
33. Chou R, Gordon DB, de Leon-Casasola OA, et al. Management of Postoperative pain: a clinical practice guideline from the american pain society, the American society of regional anesthesia and pain medicine, and the American society of anesthesiologists' committee on regional anesthesia, executive committee, and administrative council. J Pain 2016;17(2):131–57.
34. Webb CA, Mariano ER. Best multimodal analgesic protocol for total knee arthroplasty. Pain Manag 2015;5(3):185–96.
35. Kim TW, Mariano ER. Updated guide to billing for regional anesthesia (United States). Int Anesthesiol Clin 2011;49(3):84–93.
36. National correct coding initiative policy manual for medicare services – effective January 1, 2018. 2018. Available at: https://www.cms.gov/Medicare/Coding/NationalCorrectCodInitEd/index.html. Accessed December 2, 2017.
37. American Medical Association. Current Procedural Terminology (CPT) 2018 Professional Edition. Chicago: American Medical Association; 2018.
38. Sun E, Dexter F, Macario A. Can an acute pain service be cost-effective? Anesth Analg 2010;111(4):841–4.
39. Stadler M, Schlander M, Braeckman M, et al. A cost-utility and cost-effectiveness analysis of an acute pain service. J Clin Anesth 2004;16(3):159–67.
40. Lee A, Chan SK, Chen PP, et al. The costs and benefits of extending the role of the acute pain service on clinical outcomes after major elective surgery. Anesth Analg 2010;111(4):1042–50.
41. Ilfeld BM, Mariano ER, Williams BA, et al. Hospitalization costs of total knee arthroplasty with a continuous femoral nerve block provided only in the hospital versus on an ambulatory basis: a retrospective, case-control, cost-minimization analysis. Reg Anesth Pain Med 2007;32(1):46–54.
42. Brodner G, Mertes N, Buerkle H, et al. Acute pain management: analysis, implications and consequences after prospective experience with 6349 surgical patients. Eur J Anaesthesiol 2000;17(9):566–75.
43. Owen H, McMillan V, Rogowski D. Postoperative pain therapy: a survey of patients' expectations and their experiences. Pain 1990;41(3):303–7.
44. Mariano ER, Harrison TK, Kim TE, et al. Evaluation of a standardized program for training practicing anesthesiologists in ultrasound-guided regional anesthesia skills. J Ultrasound Med 2015;34(10):1883–93.
45. Udani AD, Harrison TK, Mariano ER, et al. Comparative-effectiveness of simulation-based deliberate practice versus self-guided practice on resident anesthesiologists' acquisition of ultrasound-guided regional anesthesia skills. Reg Anesth Pain Med 2016;41(2):151–7.

46. Oldman M, McCartney CJ, Leung A, et al. A survey of orthopedic surgeons' attitudes and knowledge regarding regional anesthesia. Anesth Analg 2004; 98(5):1486–90. Table of contents.

47. Mariano ER. Making it work: setting up a regional anesthesia program that provides value. Anesthesiol Clin 2008;26(4):681–92, vi.

48. Casati A, Danelli G, Baciarello M, et al. A prospective, randomized comparison between ultrasound and nerve stimulation guidance for multiple injection axillary brachial plexus block. Anesthesiology 2007;106(5):992–6.

49. Chan VW, Perlas A, McCartney CJ, et al. Ultrasound guidance improves success rate of axillary brachial plexus block. Can J Anaesth 2007;54(3):176–82.

50. Mariano ER, Cheng GS, Choy LP, et al. Electrical stimulation versus ultrasound guidance for popliteal-sciatic perineural catheter insertion: a randomized controlled trial. Reg Anesth Pain Med 2009;34(5):480–5.

51. Kim TE, Ganaway T, Harrison TK, et al. Implementation of clinical practice changes by experienced anesthesiologists after simulation-based ultrasound-guided regional anesthesia training. Korean J Anesthesiol 2017;70(3):318–26.

52. Clark DJ, Schumacher MA. America's opioid epidemic: supply and demand considerations. Anesth Analg 2017;125(5):1667–74.

53. Soelberg CD, Brown RE Jr, Du Vivier D, et al. The US opioid crisis: current federal and state legal issues. Anesth Analg 2017;125(5):1675–81.

54. Pivec R, Issa K, Naziri Q, et al. Opioid use prior to total hip arthroplasty leads to worse clinical outcomes. Int Orthop 2014;38(6):1159–65.

55. Ben-Ari A, Chansky H, Rozet I. Preoperative opioid use is associated with early revision after total knee arthroplasty: a study of male patients treated in the veterans affairs system. J Bone Joint Surg Am 2017;99(1):1–9.

56. Sing DC, Barry JJ, Cheah JW, et al. Long-acting opioid use independently predicts perioperative complication in total joint arthroplasty. J Arthroplasty 2016; 31(9 Suppl):170–4.e1.

57. Cauley CE, Anderson G, Haynes AB, et al. Predictors of in-hospital postoperative opioid overdose after major elective operations: a nationally representative cohort study. Ann Surg 2017;265(4):702–8.

58. Brummett CM, Waljee JF, Goesling J, et al. New persistent opioid use after minor and major surgical procedures in US adults. JAMA Surg 2017;152(6):e170504.

59. Hill MV, McMahon ML, Stucke RS, et al. Wide variation and excessive dosage of opioid prescriptions for common general surgical procedures. Ann Surg 2017; 265(4):709–14.

60. Waljee JF, Zhong L, Hou H, et al. The use of opioid analgesics following common upper extremity surgical procedures: a national, population-based study. Plast Reconstr Surg 2016;137(2):355e–64e.

61. Vetter TR, Kain ZN. Role of the perioperative surgical home in optimizing the perioperative use of opioids. Anesth Analg 2017;125(5):1653–7.

62. Jensen TS, Stubhaug A, Breivik H. Important development: extended acute pain service for patients at high risk of chronic pain after surgery. Scand J Pain 2016;12:58–9.

63. Katz J, Weinrib A, Fashler SR, et al. The Toronto general hospital transitional pain service: development and implementation of a multidisciplinary program to prevent chronic postsurgical pain. J Pain Res 2015;8:695–702.

64. Wanderer JP, Nathan N. A home for surgical pain management: the perioperative pain service. Anesth Analg 2017;125(4):1087.

65. Blum JM, Biel SS, Hilliard PE, et al. Preoperative ultra-rapid opiate detoxification for the treatment of post-operative surgical pain. Med Hypotheses 2015;84(6): 529–31.

Perioperative Considerations for the Patient with Opioid Use Disorder on Buprenorphine, Methadone, or Naltrexone Maintenance Therapy

Thomas Kyle Harrison, MD[a],*, Howard Kornfeld, MD[b],
Anuj Kailash Aggarwal, MD[c], Anna Lembke, MD[d,e]

KEYWORDS

- Buprenorphine • Methadone • Naltrexone • Perioperative
- Multi modal pain management • Opioid use disorder • Addiction • Relapse

KEY POINTS

- Buprenorphine and methadone for the treatment of opioid use disorder (opioid addiction) should be continued in the perioperative period for most patients.
- Oral naltrexone should be discontinued 2 days before surgery and resumed once additional opioids are no longer needed.
- Extended-release injectable naltrexone is active for 28 days with peak at 7 days.
- Multimodal pain management is critical for patients on chronic opioid therapy. Regional anesthesia, ketamine, nonsteroidal anti-inflammatory drugs, acetaminophen, dexamethasone, lidocaine, magnesium, gabapentinoids, dexmedetomidine, esmolol, and mindfulness relaxation training have all been shown to reduce opioid use and decrease postoperative pain.

[a] Department of Anesthesiology, Perioperative and Pain Medicine, Stanford School of Medicine, VA Palo Alto Health Care System, 3801 Miranda Avenue (112A), Palo Alto, CA 94304, USA; [b] Pain Fellowship Program, University of California San Francisco School of Medicine, 3 Madrona Avenue, Mill Valley, CA 94941, USA; [c] Department of Anesthesiology, Perioperative and Pain Medicine, Stanford School of Medicine, 450 Broadway, Redwood City, CA 94063, USA; [d] Department of Psychiatry and Behavioral Sciences, Stanford University School of Medicine, 401 Quarry Road, Stanford, CA 94305, USA; [e] Department of Anesthesiology and Pain Medicine, Stanford University School of Medicine, 401 Quarry Road, Stanford, CA 94305, USA
* Corresponding author.
E-mail address: kyle.harrison@stanford.edu

Anesthesiology Clin 36 (2018) 345–359
https://doi.org/10.1016/j.anclin.2018.04.002
1932-2275/18/Published by Elsevier Inc.
anesthesiology.theclinics.com

INTRODUCTION

The United States is facing the worst drug crisis in US history, with more than 63,600 drug overdose deaths in 2016, almost double the deaths caused by traffic accidents or gun violence.[1] Two-thirds of drug overdose deaths are opioid related. Furthermore, overdose death is only 1 metric by which to measure the impact of the epidemic. By conservative estimates, 2.5 million people in this country are addicted to opioids (prescription and illicit), and more than 11 million people in the United States are misusing prescription opioids obtained directly or indirectly from a doctor's prescription (according to the 2016 National Survey on Drug Use and Health).[2] Prescription opioid misuse, addiction, and overdose cost the US more than $78 billion annually.

MEDICATION-ASSISTED TREATMENT OF OPIOID USE DISORDER

The Food and Drug Administration (FDA) has approved 3 medications to target opioid use disorder/addiction:

1. Methadone (generic oral and injectable forms, Dolophine, or Methadose)
2. Buprenorphine alone (generic sublingual tablets or Probuphine intradermal implant) or combined with naloxone (Suboxone, Zubsolv, Bunavail, or generic sublingual tablets)
3. Naltrexone (generic tablets, ReVia, or Vivitrol long-acting injectable form)

The first 2 fall into a category called opioid agonist treatment, because they are both long-acting opioids that are believed to decrease the physiologic cravings that drive drug-seeking behavior. The third, naltrexone, acts as a deterrent by blocking the opioid receptor, preventing other opioids from binding. It may also reset the reward pathway through an opponent process mechanism.

All 3 of these medications, methadone maintenance, buprenorphine products, and naltrexone (oral or injectable), comprise in part what is called medication-assisted treatment of opioid use disorder. Medication-assisted treatment is defined by the Substance Abuse and Mental Health Services Administration as the use of medications in combination with counseling and behavioral therapies for the treatment of substance use disorders.

Multiple placebo-controlled trials across continents and decades demonstrate the effectiveness of opioid agonist treatment (methadone and buprenorphine) in opioid use disorder.[3-5] Both methadone and buprenorphine result in significant reductions in overdose death, illicit drug use, criminal activity, and HIV and hepatitis C incidence. These treatments are also associated with improved health status and overall improved quality of life. By contrast, short-term use of opioid agonist therapy as part of a "detoxification protocol" is rarely effective.[6,7] Patients randomized to placebo withdrawal, compared with methadone or buprenorphine maintenance treatment, are 2 times to 4 times more likely to be dead at a year.[3,8]

A Cochrane meta-analysis of oral naltrexone showed no difference compared with placebo when comparing retention in treatment, use of illicit opioids, or side effects, a year after initiating treatment.[9] However, 2 recently published studies comparing injectable extended-release naltrexone (XR-NXT) to buprenorphine-naloxone found comparable rates of retention and abstinence from heroin and other illicit drugs at 12 weeks[10] and 24 weeks,[11] respectively. The latter study[11] showed that initiating patients onto injectable naltrexone was more difficult than on buprenorphine, which may have significant real-world implications, despite comparable efficacy in this study.

BUPRENORPHINE
Pharmacology

Several decades after the development of methadone, buprenorphine—a synthetic analog of the opium poppy constituent thebaine—was discovered and introduced into clinical practice in Europe in 1978 for acute and chronic pain.[12] In the United States, the FDA approved buprenorphine for (1) acute pain in 1981 as a parenteral injection; (2) opiate use disorder in 2002, as a sublingual tablet; and (3) chronic pain in 2010, as a transdermal patch. Buprenorphine is available in many different formulations, including parenteral, sublingual tablet, sublingual film, transdermal patch, mucoadhesive film, and implant.[13] In 2017, several FDA advisory committees voted to recommend approval of an additional dose form, once-monthly and once-weekly injections of a depot form of buprenorphine for the treatment of opioid use disorder.

Although prescribing buprenorphine for addiction requires special registration (Drug Enforcement Agency Prescriber identification number X), any physician with a Drug Enforcement Agency license can prescribe it for pain. Buprenorphine retains abuse liability and thus is a Schedule III controlled drug. The range of buprenorphine doses is more than 2 orders of magnitude, with the lowest dose of the mucoadhesive form (Belbuca) at 0.075 mg (75 µg) and the highest dose of the sublingual film (Suboxone) at 12 mg (12,000 µg). This reflects the potency of low-dose forms of buprenorphine for pain, particularly in patients who are not opioid dependent, compared with the higher doses used for patients with opioid use disorder. The high-dose forms of buprenorphine are available as a monoproduct containing only buprenorphine but also in a form combined with naloxone in a 4:1 ratio. The addition of naloxone helps prevent misuse because it induces withdrawal symptoms when injected intravenously (IV).

Buprenorphine is unique in that it acts as both an agonist and antagonist at different opioid receptors. Buprenorphine has a high binding affinity at the mu receptor but only partially activates it compared with other opioids. Despite partial activation, buprenorphine still provides analgesia but has a ceiling effect on respiratory depression, conferring significantly less risk of respiratory compromise and overdose compared with opioids, such as morphine and fentanyl.[14] Unique to buprenorphine is its antagonism of the kappa opioid receptor, which, along with its agonist action at the nociceptin opioid receptor (ORL-1), may confer several advantages over other opioids. These advantages include improved respiratory safety and attenuated euphoria and may contribute to its role in managing neuropathic pain, opioid-induced hyperalgesia, and psychiatric syndromes.[15]

As a result of its extensive first-pass metabolism, oral bioavailability is poor and buprenorphine is often given via the sublingual (or transmucosal) routes. Due to its lipophilic nature and potency, buprenorphine is remarkably well suited to transdermal delivery.

Respiratory depression can occur when buprenorphine is used along with central nervous system sedating agents, including alcohol, sedative-hypnotics, and neuroleptic drugs, or in fragile, young, or elderly populations. Reversal requires greater than the usual dose of naloxone: a 2-mg bolus is usually recommended in adults followed by 4-mg per hour infusion under close observation.[16]

Buprenorphine is primarily metabolized in the liver by phase I reactions (N-dealkylation) through the cytochrome P450 Cyp 3A4 enzyme to norbuprenorhpine. Both buprenorphine and norbuprenorphine are conjugated by uridine 5′ diphosphoglucuronosyltransferase (UGT), in phase II reactions to their glucuronide forms. Buprenorphine and norbuprenorphine are primarily eliminated through bile and feces. Only a small amount of the glucuronide metabolites are excreted in the kidney. These pharmacokinetics confer relative safety compared with other opioids, when buprenorphine is used in patients with moderate to severe hepatic failure or in renal insufficiency. Due to little influence of buprenorphine on the activity of the cytochrome p450 Cyp 3A4 enzyme, drug-drug interactions are usually not a significant concern.[17]

Due to its tight binding and attenuated intrinsic activity at the mu receptor, parenteral or sublingual (but not transdermal) buprenorphine can precipitate withdrawal symptoms in patients who are dependent on other opioids. Therefore, an induction process involving early opioid withdrawal before introduction of sublingual buprenorphine is required.

Perioperative Use

Buprenorphine's ability to tightly bind to the mu receptor and potentially block additional opioids from binding has created a concern that additional opioids are less effective in the presence of buprenorphine, thus reducing the analgesic efficacy. Clinical research conducted early in the history of buprenorphine development[18] and multiple investigations and clinical practice in more recent years,[19,20] however, provide strong reassurance that standard opioids given to buprenorphine maintained patients are effective and additive to the baseline analgesia associated with the buprenorphine.

Clinical guidelines issued in 2004 by the Center for Substance Abuse Treatment,[21] despite acknowledging lack of evidence, set into motion a misconception in the United States, widely quoted, that perioperative analgesia is difficult to achieve with standard opioids in buprenorphine-maintained patients and that buprenorphine in most cases should be stopped and converted to methadone preoperatively. This misunderstanding may stem from addiction research, which did not assess analgesia but rather demonstrated that buprenorphine in higher doses blocked the euphoric and reinforcing effects of subsequently administered heroin.[22]

Case studies have been published describing difficult to control pain in postoperative buprenorphine-maintained patients.[23,24] Other cases, however, have been published describing adequate management, particularly when combined with multimodal analgesia.[22,25]

Extenuating circumstances, including intraoperative nerve injury, nonoptimal dosing of buprenorphine, and failure to use multimodal analgesia in a timely way characterize the published cases reporting difficult postoperative analgesia.[22] Furthermore, difficult postoperative analgesia is a common occurrence in patients who are preoperatively dependent on opioids of any type.

The experience in Australia established opioids were effective in hospitalized and postsurgical patients maintained on buprenorphine.[26,27] This was confirmed by US obstetricians, who did discontinue buprenorphine in pregnant patients for either vaginal deliveries or planned caesarean sections and reported adequate pain control.[28–30]

Stopping buprenorphine in stabilized opioid use disorder and/or chronic pain patients confers medical risk, discomfort, and logistical burden on patients, their prescribing clinicians, and the health system. A significant opioid debt will exist that will need to be filled with another opioid, risking over-dosing or under-dosing, and reinduction can be clinically and symptomatically problematic in the immediate postoperative period and can also prolong hospital stays.

Optimal use of buprenorphine in the perioperative setting has not be established. Whether to continue a patient's current dose or wean the dose down but not off to provide more mu receptor availability has not been studied. Nonetheless, receptor binding studies using radiolabeled carfentanil and PET scans to identify available mu receptors in buprenorphine-treated heroin-addicted persons confirm a dose-response curve of reduced but conserved receptors available for additional analgesia, even at high sublingual doses of buprenorphine.[31] Which opioid to use for additional analgesia has not been studied, but using opioids that have higher mu receptor affinity, such as sufentanil, fentanyl, or hydromorphone, should be considered. Increasing the buprenorphine as the primary opioid analgesic has also been advocated by some investigators as well as dividing the daily dose into 3-times-daily dosing because a daily dose may not provide adequate analgesia throughout the entire 24-hour period.[32,33] Finally, patients who have stopped buprenorphine postoperatively and are still taking additional opioids potentially could be restarted on buprenorphine by using a daily microdose escalation known as the Bernese method without precipitating withdrawal. Once a sufficient dose of buprenorphine is reached, patients can discontinue their additional postoperative opioids.[34]

METHADONE
Pharmacology

Methadone is a full mu opioid receptor agonist. It is a racemic mixture with the R enantiomer responsible for the opioid effect and the R and S enantiomers having N-methyl-D-aspartate receptor (NMDA) antagonist activity. Oral administration has a moderate bioavailability approximately of 70% to 80% and is 90% bound to plasma proteins. Peak plasma levels are reached within 2 hours to 4 hours. Methadone undergoes a biphasic pattern of elimination—α-elimination (8–12 hours) and β-elimination (30–60 hours). The α-elimination is associated with analgesia and the β-elimination with withdrawal suppression. Methadone is metabolized in the liver and eliminated through renal and fecal routes. Hepatic metabolism is through the cytochrome P450 system, and coadministered medications that induce or inhibit the cytochrome P450 system can dramatically alter the metabolism, resulting in lower or higher systemic levels for the same dose of methadone. Methadone binds approximately 30% of the mu receptors allowing for additional activity from both endogenous and exogenous mu opioid agonists.[35,36]

Sedation, respiratory depression, and death can occur with increasing doses of methadone. The toxic dose can be difficult to predict secondary to long half-life, changes in metabolism, and variable tolerance profile at higher doses. Methadone can also increase the OT interval and has been associated with sudden cardiac death. Prolongation of the QT to greater than 500 milliseconds is associated with arrhythmias, including torsades de pointes.[37]

Perioperative Use

Patients should take their usual dose of methadone on the day of surgery. Patients are opioid tolerant; thus, additional opioids likely are needed. Patients should be continued on their home maintenance dose throughout the perioperative period. Because the α-elimination (8 hours) is associated with the analgesic component of methadone, dosing a patient's daily dose in 3 divided doses might improve pain control.[38] It is important to confirm a patient's home dose with the methadone prescriber. If there is concern about what the actual dose is, the methadone can be administered in divided doses throughout the day, monitoring for sedation and respiratory depression. Patients unable to take their oral dose should be given IV methadone. The IV dose should be reduced by one-half to two-thirds and be given in divided dose every 6 hours to 8 hours. Oral to IV conversion can be difficult, especially at higher doses, so consulting with a pharmacist or the methadone prescriber may be warranted. Up-titration of methadone in the perioperative period is not advised secondary to the long half-life. If any up-titration occurs, it should be in consultation with a patient's methadone prescriber or expert on the use of methadone. If a patient's methadone dose has been interrupted for more than 5 days, restarting should be in consultation with a provider who is experienced in methadone maintenance induction.[39] Documenting the contact number of the methadone prescriber is important so appropriate follow-up at discharge can be arranged.

NALTREXONE
Pharmacology

Naltrexone is a semisynthetic opioid antagonist derived from oxymorphone via substitution of the N-methyl group with metylcyclopropyl group. It is a competitive antagonist at mu opioid receptors and partial agonist at kappa receptors and has minimal activity at delta receptors.[40] In oral formulation, it has rapid absorption, with peak concentration at 1 hour, undergoing first-pass hepatic metabolism.[41] After continuous administration for 7 days, the half-life is approximately 10 hours with renal excretion.[42] XR-NXT, a biodegradable microsphere matrix embedded with naltrexone, was introduced in 2010 as a 380-mg gluteal intramuscular injection to yield opioid antagonism for 28 days.[42] Pharmacokinetically, XR-NXT peaks at 7 days and avoids first-pass hepatic metabolism.[43] Opioid antagonist effects of XR-NXT decrease over the course of a month. Although currently there are no published data determining exactly when opioid antagonism can be overcome, case reports suggest it can be achieved during the fourth week postinjection.[44]

Perioperative Use

With a 10-hour half-life, oral naltrexone should be discontinued approximately 2–3 days before surgery in close coordination with the patient and prescribing physician, accounting for 5 half-lives. For XR-NXT, there is less guidance; however, a balanced risk-benefit decision of need for surgery and ability to use opioid-sparing techniques, including regional and neuraxial anesthetics, needs to be considered. Successful pain management has been reported starting in the fourth week of treatment, with complete lack of analgesia to opioids in the first 2 weeks of treatment.[43,44] Close monitoring may be required, however, if patients receive opioids postoperatively because variable responses have been observed, including both attenuation and enhancement; in some animal studies, levels 6 times to 20 times typical doses of opioids have been needed to achieve analgesia.[45–47] Restarting naltrexone requires patients to be free of opioids to avoid acute withdrawal. FDA-approved prescribing information advises patients to be abstinent from opioids for 7 days to 10 days prior to induction.[48]

MULTIMODAL PAIN MANAGEMENT

Multimodal pain management is important to improve efficacy and minimize side effects. Multimodal therapies are even more important for the opioid use disorder patient because these patients are opioid tolerant but often pain intolerant (**Table 1**).

Table 1
Multimodal pain management

Opioids	Acetaminophen	Gabapentinoids
Regional anesthesia	Dexamethasone (>0.1 mg/kg)	Dexmedetomidine
Ketamine	Lidocaine infusion	Esmolol
NSAIDs	Magnesium infusion	Mindfulness relaxation

Opioids

Opioids are still an important component of multimodal pain management; however, doses need to be increased in opioid-tolerant patients. The degree of tolerance can be difficult to predict and patients are still at risk for respiratory depression from increasing doses of opioids. Continuing the preoperative dose of opioids is important to prevent withdrawal. Early withdrawal is subjective and often results in increased pain, but as it progresses physical signs of withdrawal become evident (sweating, gastrointestinal upset, tremor, restlessness, anxiety, yawning, gooseflesh, and runny nose/tearing). As with all patients receiving perioperative opioids, careful monitoring for sedation and respiratory depression is critical.[49,50]

Regional Anesthesia

Regional anesthesia is vital to anesthetic management of opioid-tolerant patients. Neuraxial anesthesia or use of peripheral nerve blocks reduces both pain and opioid requirements and improves patient satisfaction.[51–53] Single-injection spinal with opioid (morphine or hydromorphone) with or without local anesthetic has been associated with lower pain and decreased systemic opioid requirements.[54] Thoracic epidural anesthesia is associated with decreased pain and reduced opioid requirements.[55] Transversus abdominis plane blocks provide superior pain control and lower opioid requirements for abdominal surgery compared with opioids alone.[56–58] Continuous peripheral nerve blockade is associated with improved pain control, lower opioid requirements, and greater patient satisfaction compared with single injection.[59]

Ketamine

Ketamine is an IV anesthetic and NMDA receptor antagonist. It has been shown to improve postoperative pain control as well as decrease opioid consumption in both opioid-naïve and opioid-tolerant patients. Several different dosing protocols have been studied but low-dose ketamine (0–1 mg/kg bolus and infusion of <1.2 mg/kg/h) is safe and effective at reducing both opioid consumption and time to first opioid request.[60,61] Ketamine administered at 0.5 mg/kg IV at induction and at an infusion of 10 µg/kg/min until skin closure decreased both reported pain scores as well as morphine consumption in opioid-tolerant patients at 48 hours and at 6 weeks.[62] One case report suggests potential for ketamine misuse and addiction when initiated as an analgesic alternative in a patient with opioid use disorder on buprenorphine.[63]

Lidocaine

Perioperative use of lidocaine has been shown to reduce pain scores and opioid use in the immediate postoperative period up to 24 hours. The analgesic effects were most apparent after laparoscopic and open abdominal surgery. It has also been shown to reduce ileus, postoperative nausea and vomiting, and hospital length of stay. Common dosing for perioperative lidocaine infusion is 1.5 mg/kg/h to 3 mg/kg/h after a bolus of 0 mg/kg IV to 1.5 mg/kg IV. It can be run in the immediate postoperative period usually at a lower dose. There are no data for use greater than 24 hours. Lidocaine has a narrow therapeutic index, with therapeutic levels occurring at 2.5 µg/mL to 3.5 µg/mL but with central nervous system toxicity occurring at 5 µg/kg and cardiovascular toxicity at 10 µg/mL. Lidocaine toxicity should be treated 20% lipid emulsion and supportive care.[64–67]

Magnesium

Magnesium is an often overlooked adjunct in acute pain management. A meta-analysis of 1200 patients showed IV magnesium reduced both early and late pain at rest and late pain with movement. Magnesium has also been shown to have a large effect on reducing perioperative opioid use. The usual dose range is 30-mg/kg to 50-mg/kg bolus followed by a 10-mg/kg infusion intraoperatively. Several studies continued the infusion for 24 hours to 48 hours at a reduced rate. Continuing the infusion may provide additional benefit compared withw intraoperative use only.[68] Magnesium may also help prevent opioid-induced hyperalgesia.[69]

Acetaminophen

Acetaminophen can be administered orally, rectally, or IV. The exact mechanism of action is unknown but it is believed to inhibit cyclooxygenase (COX) enzyme in the central nervous system.[70] A meta-analysis showed that 36% of patients receiving IV acetaminophen experienced at least a 50% reduction in pain and used 26% less opioids in the first 4 hours postoperatively.[71] Oral and IV administration seem to have similar efficacy.[72] Combining acetaminophen with nonsteroidal anti-inflammatory drugs (NSAIDs) confers additional analgesic efficacy over either drug alone.[73]

Gabapentinoids

Gabapentinoids (gabapentin and pregabalin) are a class of drug that bind to the $\alpha2\delta$ subunit of the voltage-dependent calcium channel, thus inhibiting the opening of the calcium channel and reducing release of excitatory neurotransmitters. Gabapentin and pregabalin have been shown to reduce postoperative pain and reduce opioid consumption; however, they have been associated with an increase in sedation and dizziness.[74,75] When gabapentin was added to a methadone[76] or buprenorphine-assisted detoxification program, it reduced withdrawal symptoms.[77]

Nonsteroidal Anti-inflammatory Drugs

Nonselective NSAIDs (eg, ibuprofen, naproxen, and ketorolac) inhibit both the COX-1 and COX-2 isoforms whereas celecoxib is selective for the COX-2 isoform. COX inhibitors decrease conversion of arachidonic acid to prostaglandins and thromboxane, thus reducing pain and inflammation. NSAIDs have been shown to reduce pain and decrease opioid use postoperatively. Caution should be used in patients with cardiovascular disease, renal insufficiency, and gastrointestinal bleeding. The risk is increased with long term use however the risk of brief postoperative use is unclear.[70,78–81]

Steroids

Dexamethasone is a corticosteroid that has been shown to reduce pain and opioid use. A meta-analysis of 2500 patients showed that intermediate dose of dexamethasone (0.11–0.2 mg/kg) had opioid-sparing effects as well as reduced early and late pain at rest and movement. Low dose (less than 0.1 mg/kg) was not effective. Dexamethasone is more efficacious if it is administered preoperatively. Rapid administration of a small volume of dexamethasone can cause perineal pain. This risk can be reduced by giving the dose over 10 minutes and in a larger volume (50 mL). Wound infections or delayed wound healing did not seem associated with the intermediate dose. The risk-benefit analysis of perioperative blood glucose control versus pain control should be considered. The effects on blood glucose were not addressed in the meta-analysis.[82]

Dexmedetomidine

Dexmedetomidine is an α_2-adrenergic receptor agonist, which has sedative, anxiolytic, sympatholytic, and analgesic properties. When used intraoperatively, it can reduce the need for opioids and decreases pain intensity. The degree of opioid sparing is stronger than acetaminophen but weaker than ketamine or NSAIDs. Dexmedetomidine can cause hypotension and bradycardia.[83–85]

Esmolol

Esmolol is an ultra–short-acting β_1-receptor antagonist. It has been shown to decrease intraoperative and postoperative opioid consumption when used intraoperatively.[86]

Table 2
Medication-assisted treatment of opioid use disorder: perioperative considerations

Drug	Preoperative	Day of Surgery	Postoperative
Buprenorphine	Continue daily dose. Document buprenorphine provider's contact information for postoperative follow-up.	Patient should receive usual daily dose. Plan for multimodal pain management.	Continue daily dose but consider switching to TID dosing. Consider increasing buprenorphine to target pain. Continue multimodal pain management. Arrange for follow-up with buprenorphine provider early in the postoperative period. Discharge with the lowest dose and shortest duration of additional opioids as possible.
Methadone	Continue daily dose. Document methadone dose and methadone provider's contact information for postoperative follow-up.	Patient should receive usual daily dose. If unable to take PO, give IV (reduce dose by 1/2 to 2/3 and split into TID dosing). Plan for multimodal pain management.	Continue daily dose but consider switching to TID dosing. Continue multimodal pain management. Arrange for follow-up with methadone provider early in the postoperative period. If daily dosing patient may need to go to methadone clinic postoperatively. Discharge with the lowest dose and shortest duration of additional opioids as possible
Naltrexone	Oral—discontinue >48 h preoperatively. XR-NXT—discontinue 30 d preoperatively.	Confirm last dose >48 h for oral and >30 d for implanted XR-NXT. Plan for multimodal pain management.	Continue multimodal pain management. Patient may be more sensitive to opioids. Resume after patient has been off opioids for 7 d.

Psychological

Psychological factors affecting pain include general anxiety, depression, posttraumatic stress disorder, pain-related anxiety, and pain catastrophizing.[87] A single scripted 15-minute session of mindfulness training or hypnotic suggestion delivered in a hospital setting has been shown to reduce pain intensity by up to 30% in one-third of patients who were reporting severe pain. Preoperatively addressing a patient's risk of pain catastrophizing can also help decrease postoperative pain.[88]

SUMMARY

The appropriate use of buprenorphine, methadone, and naltrexone in the perioperative period, for patients with opioid use disorder on maintenance therapy, is an increasingly important part of modern medical treatment (**Table 2**). Buprenorphine and methadone should be continued in the perioperative period for most patients. Oral naltrexone should be discontinued 2 days before surgery and resumed once additional opioids are no longer needed. Multimodal pain management is critical for patients on chronic opioid therapy. Regional anesthesia, ketamine, NSAIDs, acetaminophen, dexamethasone, lidocaine, magnesium, gabapentinoids, dexmedetomidine, esmolol, and mindfulness relaxation training have all been shown to reduce opioid use and decrease postoperative pain.

ACKNOWLEDGMENTS

Dr H. Kornfeld would like to acknowledge Heidi Molga, BS, for her research and editorial assistance in contributing to this work.

REFERENCES

1. Hedegaard H, Warner M, Minino AM. Drug overdose deaths in the United States, 1999-2016. In: NCHS Data Brief No.294, 2017. Available at: https://www.cdc.gov/nchs/products/databriefs/db294.htm. Accessed January 8, 2018.
2. Center for Behavioral Health Statistics and Quality. 2016 national survey on drug use and health: detailed tables. Rockville (MD): Substance Abuse and Mental Health Services Administration; 2017.
3. Sordo L, Barrio G, Bravo MJ, et al. Mortality risk during and after opioid substitution treatment: systematic review and meta-analysis of cohort studies. BMJ 2017; 357:j1550.
4. Nielsen S, Larance B, Degenhardt L, et al. Opioid agonist treatment for pharmaceutical opioid dependent people. Cochrane Database Syst Rev 2016;(5):CD011117.
5. Mattick RP, Breen C, Kimber J, et al. Buprenorphine maintenance versus placebo or methadone maintenance for opioid dependence. Cochrane Database Syst Rev 2014;(2):CD002207.
6. Amato L, Davoli M, Minozzi S, et al. Methadone at tapered doses for the management of opioid withdrawal. Cochrane Database Syst Rev 2013;(2):CD003409.
7. Dunn KE, Sigmon SC, Strain EC, et al. The association between outpatient buprenorphine detoxification duration and clinical treatment outcomes: a review. Drug Alcohol Depend 2011;119(1–2):1–9.
8. Strang J, Babor T, Caulkins J, et al. Drug policy and the public good: evidence for effective interventions. Lancet 2012;379(9810):71–83.
9. Lobmaier P, Kornor H, Kunoe N, et al. Sustained-release naltrexone for opioid dependence. Cochrane Database Syst Rev 2008;(2):CD006140.

10. Tanum L, Solli K, Latif Z, et al. The effectiveness of injectable extended-release naltrexone vs daily buprenorphine-naloxone for opioid dependence: a randomized clinical noninferiority trial. JAMA Psychiatry 2017;74(12):1197–205.
11. Lee JD, Nunes EV Jr, Novo P, et al. Comparative effectiveness of extended-release naltrexone versus buprenorphine-naloxone for opioid relapse prevention (X: BOT): a multicentre, open-label, randomized controlled trial. Lancet 2018; 391(10118):309–18.
12. Johnson RE, Fudala PJ, Payne R. Buprenorphine: considerations for pain management. J Pain Symptom Manage 2005;29:297–326.
13. Center for Drug Evaluation and Research (U.S.). Orange book: approved drug products with therapeutic equivalence evaluations. 37th edition. Rockville (MD): U.S. Dept. of Health and Human Services, Food and Drug Administration, Center for Drug Evaluation and Research, Office of Pharmaceutical Science, Office of Generic Drugs; 2017.
14. Raffa RB, Haidery M, Huang HM, et al. The clinical analgesic efficacy of buprenorphine. J Clin Pharm Ther 2014;39(6):577–83.
15. Davis MP. Twelve reasons for considering buprenorphine as a frontline analgesic in the management of pain. J Support Oncol 2012;10:209–19.
16. Dahan A. New insights into buprenorphine's respiratory effects. In: Budd K, Raffa RB, editors. Buprenorphine- the unique opioid analgesic. New York: Thieme; 2005. p. 22–32.
17. Walsh SL, Middleton LS. Buprenorphine pharmacodynamics and pharmacokinetics. In: Cruciani RA, Knotkova H, editors. Handbook of methadone prescribing and buprenorphine therapy. New York: Springer; 2013. p. 163–81.
18. Atkinson RE, Schofield P, Mellor P. The efficacy in sequential use of buprenorphine and morphine in advanced cancer pain. In: Doyle D, editor. Opioids in the treatment of cancer pain: proceedings of a symposium sponsored by Reckitt & Colman Pharmaceuticals and held at the Royal College of Surgeons, London. International congress and symposium series, 146. London: Royal Society of Medicine Services Limited; 1990. p. 81–7.
19. Mercadante S, Villari P, Ferrera P, et al. Safety and effectiveness of intravenous morphine for episodic breakthrough pain in patients receiving transdermal buprenorphine. J Pain Symptom Manage 2006;32:175–9.
20. Van Niel JCG, Schneider J, Tzschentke TM. Efficacy of full μ-opioid receptor agonists is not impaired by concomitant buprenorphine or mixed opioid agonists/antagonists–preclinical and clinical evidence. Drug Res (Stuttg) 2016;66(11): 562–70.
21. Center for Substance Abuse Treatment. Clinical guidelines for the use of buprenorphine in the treatment of opioid addiction. Treatment Improvement Protocol (TIP) Series 40. DHHS Publication No. (SMA) 04–3939. Rockville (MD): Substance Abuse and Mental Health Services Administration; 2004.
22. Silvia MJ, Rubinstein A. Continuous perioperative sublingual buprenorphine. J Pain Palliat Care Pharmacother 2016;30(4):289–93.
23. Huang A, Katznelson R, de Perrot M, et al. Perioperative management of a patient undergoing Clagett window closure stabilized on suboxone for chronic pain: a case report. Can J Anaesth 2014;61:826–31.
24. McCormick Z, Chu SK, Chang-Chien GC, et al. Acute pain control challenges with buprenorphine/naloxone therapy in a patient with compartment syndrome secondary to McArdle's disease: a case report and review. Pain Med 2013;14: 1187–91.

25. Kornfeld H, Manfredi L. Effectiveness of full agonist opioids in patients stabilized on buprenorphine undergoing major surgery: a case series. Am J Ther 2010;17: 523–8.
26. Roberts DM, Meyer-Witting M. High-dose buprenorphine: perioperative precautions and management strategies. Anaesth Intensive Care 2005;33:17–25.
27. Macintyre PE, Russell RA, Usher KAN, et al. Pain relief and opioid requirements in the first 24 h after surgery in patients taking buprenorphine and methadone opioid substitution therapy. Anaesth Intensive Care 2013;41:222–30.
28. Meyer M, Paranya G, Norris AK, et al. Intrapartum and postpartum analgesia for women maintained on buprenorphine during pregnancy. Eur J Pain 2010;14(9): 939–43.
29. Vilkins AL, Bagley SM, Hahn KA, et al. Comparison of post-cesarean section opioid analgesic requirements in women with opioid use disorder treated with methadone or buprenorphine. J Addict Med 2017;11(5):397–401.
30. Leighton BL, Crock LW. Case series of successful postoperative pain management in buprenorphine maintenance therapy patients. Anesth Analg 2017; 125(5):1779–83.
31. Greenwald MK, Johanson CE, Moody DE, et al. Effects of buprenorphine maintenance dose on mu-opioid receptor availability, plasma concentrations, and antagonist blockade in heroin-dependent volunteers. Neuropsychopharmacology 2003;28:2000–9.
32. Anderson TA, Quaye ANA, Ward N, et al. To stop or not, that is the question-acute pain management for the patient on chronic buprenorphine. Anesth Analg 2017; 126(6):1180–6.
33. Childers JW, Arnold RM. Treatment of pain in patients taking buprenorphine for opioid addiction #221. J Palliat Med 2012;15(5):613–4.
34. Hammig R, Kemter A, Strasser J, et al. Use of microdose for induction of buprenorphine treatment with overlapping full opioid agonist use: the Bernese method. Subst Abuse Rehabil 2016;7:99–105.
35. Kling MA, Carson RE, Borg L, et al. Opioid receptor imaging with positron emission tomography and [(18)F]cyclofoxy in long-term, methadone-treated former heroin addicts. J Pharmacol Exp Ther 2000;295:1070–6.
36. McCance-Katz EF, Sullivan LE, Nallani S. Drug interactions of clinical importance among the opioids, methadone and buprenorphine, and other frequently prescribed medications: a review. Am J Addict 2010;19:4–16.
37. Martin JA, Campbell A, Killip T, et al. QT interval screening in methadone maintenance treatment: report of a SAMHSA expert panel. J Addict Dis 2011;30(4): 283–306.
38. Peng PWH, Tumber PS, Gourlay D. Perioperative pain management of patients on methadone therapy. Can J Anaesth 2005;52:513.
39. Methadone maintenance treatment program standards and clinical guidelines. 2011. Available at: http://www.cpso.on.ca/uploadedFiles/members/MMT-Guidelines. pdf. Accessed December 18, 2017.
40. Wentland MP, Lou R, Lu Q, et al. Syntheses of novel high affinity ligands for opioid receptors. Bioorg Med Chem Lett 2009;19(8):2289–94.
41. Wall ME, Brine DR, Perez-Reyes M. The metabolismof naltrexone in man. NIDA Res Monogr 1981;28:105–31.
42. Sudakin D. Naltrexone: not just for opioids anymore. J Med Toxicol 2016;12:71–5.
43. Dunbar JL, Turncliff RZ, Dong Q, et al. Single- and multiple-dose pharmacokinetics of long acting injectable naltrexone. Alcohol Clin Exp Res 2006;30(3): 480–90.

44. Curatolo C, Trinh M. Challenges in the perioperative management of the patient receiving extended-release naltrexone. A A Case Rep 2014;3:142–4.
45. Dean RL, Todtenkopf MS, Deaver DR, et al. Overriding the blockade of antinociceptive actions of opioids in rats treated with extended-release naltrexone. Pharmacol Biochem Behav 2008;89:515–22.
46. Díaz A, Pazos A, Flórez J, et al. Regulation of mu-opioid receptors, G-protein-coupled receptor kinases and beta-arrestin 2 in the rat brain after chronic opioid receptor antagonism. Neuroscience 2002;112:345–53.
47. Tempel A, Gardner EL, Zukin RS. Neurochemical and functional correlates of naltrexone-induced opiate receptor up-regulation. J Pharmacol Exp Ther 1985; 232:439–44.
48. Sigmon SC, Bisaga A, Nunes EV, et al. Opioid detoxification and naltrexone induction strategies: recommendations for clinical practice. Am J Drug Alcohol Abuse 2012;38(3):187–99.
49. Huxtable CA, Roberts LJ, Somogyi AA, et al. Acute pain management in opioid-tolerant patients: a growing challenge. Anaesth Intensive Care 2011;39(5): 804–23.
50. Shah S, Kapoor S, Durkin B. Analgesic management of acute pain in the opioid-tolerant patient. Curr Opin Anaesthesiol 2015;28(4):398–402.
51. Kumar K, Kirksey MA, Duong S, et al. A review of opioid-sparing modalities in perioperative pain management: methods to decrease opioid use postoperatively. Anesth Analg 2017;125(5):1749–60.
52. Richman JM, Liu SS, Courpas G, et al. Does continuous peripheral nerve block provide superior pain control to opioids? A meta-analysis. Anesth Analg 2006; 102:248–57.
53. Liu SS, Strodtbeck WM, Richman JM, et al. A comparison of regional versus general anesthesia for ambulatory anesthesia: a meta-analysis of randomized controlled trials. Anesth Analg 2005;101:1634–42.
54. Meylan N, Elia N, Lysakowski C, et al. Benefit and risk of intrathecal morphine without local anaesthetic in patients undergoing major surgery: meta-analysis of randomized trials. Br J Anaesth 2009;102(2):156–67.
55. Block BM, Liu SS, Rowlingson AJ, et al. Efficacy of postoperative epidural analgesia: a meta-analysis. JAMA 2003;290(18):2455–63.
56. Baeriswyl M, Kirkham KR, Kern C, et al. The analgesic efficacy of ultrasound-guided transversus abdominis plane block in adult patients: a meta-analysis. Anesth Analg 2015;121(6):1640–54.
57. McEvoy M, Scott MJ, Gordon DB, et al. American Society for Enhanced Recovery (ASER) and Perioperative Quality Initiative (POQI) joint consensus statement on optimal analgesia within an enhanced recovery pathway for colorectal surgery: part 1-from the preoperative period to PACU. Perioper Med (Lond) 2017;6:8.
58. McEvoy M, Scott MJ, Gordon DB, et al. American Society for Enhanced Recovery (ASER) and Perioperative Quality Initiative (POQI) joint consensus statement on optimal analgesia within an enhanced recovery pathway for colorectal surgery: part 2-from PACU to the transition home. Perioper Med 2017;6:7.
59. Bingham AE, Fu R, Horn JL, et al. Continuous peripheral nerve block compared with single-injection peripheral nerve block a systematic review and meta-analysis of randomized controlled trials. Reg Anesth Pain Med 2012;37:583–94.
60. De Oliveira GS, Benzon HT, White PF. The role of nonopioid analgesic infusions in the management of postoperative pain. In: Hadzic A, editor. Hadzic's textbook of regional anesthesia and acute pain management. 2nd edition. New York: McGraw-Hill; 2017. p. 1226–37.

61. Laskowski K, Stirling A, McKay WP, et al. A systematic review of intravenous ketamine for postoperative analgesia. Can J Anaesth 2011;58(10):911–23.
62. Loftus RW, Yeager MP, Clark JA, et al. Intraoperative ketamine reduces perioperative opiate consumption in opiate-dependent patients with chronic back pain undergoing back surgery. Anesthesiology 2010;113:639–46.
63. Prekupec MP, Sussman RS, Sher Y, et al. Relapse on ketamine followed by severe and prolonged withdrawal. J Nat Sci 2017;3(10):1–4.
64. Kranke P, Jokinen J, Pace NL, et al. Continuous intravenous perioperative lidocaine infusion for postoperative pain and recovery. Cochrane Database Syst Rev 2015;(7):CD009642.
65. Eipe N, Gupta S, Penning J. Intravenous lidocaine for acute pain: an evidence-based clinical update. BJA Educ 2016;16(9):292–8.
66. Weibel S, Jokinen J, Pace NL, et al. Efficacy and safety of intravenous lidocaine for postoperative analgesia and recovery after surgery: a systematic review with trial sequential analysis. Br J Anaesth 2016;116(6):770–83.
67. Dunn LK, Durieux ME. Perioperative use of intravenous lidocaine. Anesthesiology 2017;126(4):729–37.
68. De Oliveira GS Jr, Castro-Alves LJ, Khan JH, et al. Perioperative systemic magnesium to minimize postoperative pain: a meta-analysis of randomized controlled trials. Anesthesiology 2013;119:178–90.
69. Song JW, Lee YW, Yoon KB, et al. Magnesium sulfate prevents remifentanil-induced postoperative hyperalgesia in patients undergoing thyroidectomy. Anesth Analg 2011;113(2):390–7.
70. Young AC, Buvanendran A. Multimodal analgesia: pharmacologic interventions and prevention of persistent postoperative pain. In: Hadzic A, editor. Hadzic's textbook of regional anesthesia and acute pain management. 2nd edition. New York: McGraw-Hill; 2017. p. 1219–26.
71. McNicol ED, Ferguson MC, Haroutounian S, et al. Single dose intravenous paracetamol or intravenous propacetamol for postoperative pain. Cochrane Database Syst Rev 2016;(5):CD007126.
72. Jibril F, Sharaby S, Mohamed A, et al. Intravenous versus oral acetaminophen for pain: systematic review of current evidence to support clinical decision-making. Can J Hosp Pharm 2015;68(3):238–47.
73. Kaye AD, Cornett EM, Helander E, et al. An update on nonopioids intravenous or oral analgesics for perioperative pain management. Anesthesiol Clin 2017;35: 55–71.
74. Hurley RW, Cohen SP, Williams KA, et al. The analgesic effects of perioperative gabapentin on postoperative pain: a meta-analysis. Reg Anesth Pain Med 2006;31(3):237–47.
75. Arumugam S, Lau CSM, Chamberlain RS. Use of preoperative gabapentin significantly reduces postoperative opioid consumption: a meta-analysis. J Pain Res 2016;9:631–40.
76. Moghadam MS, Alavinia M. The effects of gabapentin on methadone based addiction treatment: a randomized controlled trial. Pak J Pharm Sci 2013;26(5): 985–9.
77. Sanders NC, Mancino MJ, Gentry WB, et al. Randomized, placebo-controlled pilot trial of gabapentin during an outpatient, buprenorphine-assisted detoxification procedure. Exp Clin Psychopharmacol 2013;21(4):294–302.
78. Moore RA, Derry S, Aldington D, et al. Single dose oral analgesics for acute postoperative pain in adults - an overview of Cochrane reviews. Cochrane Database Syst Rev 2015;(9):CD008659.

79. Alexander R, El-Moalem HE, Gan TJ. Comparison of the morphine- sparing effects of diclofenac sodium and ketoroiac tromethamine after major orthopedic surgery. J Clin Anesth 2002;14:187–92.
80. Straube S, Derry S, McQuay HJ, et al. Effect of preoperative Cox-II-selective NSAIDs (coxibs) on postoperative outcomes: a systematic review of randomized studies. Acta Anaesthesiol Scand 2005;49(5):601–13.
81. De Oliveira GS Jr, Agarwal D, Benzon HT. Perioperative single dose ketorolac to prevent postoperative pain: a meta-analysis of randomized trials. Anesth Analg 2012;114(2):424–33.
82. De Oliveira GS Jr, Almeida MD, Benzon HT, et al. Perioperative single dose systemic dexamethasone for postoperative pain: a meta-analysis of randomized controlled trials. Anesthesiology 2011;115(3):575–88.
83. Tang C, Xia Z. Dexmedetomidine in perioperative acute pain management: a non-opioid adjuvant analgesic. J Pain Res 2017;11(10):1899–904.
84. Blaudszun G, Lysakowski C, Elia N, et al. Effect of perioperative systemic alpha2 agonists on postoperative morphine consumption and pain intensity: systematic review and meta-analysis of randomized controlled trials. Anesthesiology 2012;116(6):1312–22.
85. Wenzel JT, Schwenk ES, Baratta JL, et al. Managing opioid-tolerant patients in the perioperative surgical home. Anesthesiol Clin 2016;34(2):287–301.
86. Gelineau AM, King MR, Ladha KS, et al. Intraoperative esmolol as an adjunct for perioperative opioid and postoperative pain reduction: a systematic review, meta-analysis, and meta-regression. Anesth Analg 2018;126(3):1035–49.
87. Darnall BD. Pain psychology and pain catastrophizing in the perioperative setting: a review of impacts, interventions and unmet needs. Hand Clin 2016;32(1):33–9.
88. Garland EL, Baker AK, Larsen P, et al. Randomized controlled trial of brief mindfulness training and hypnotic suggestion for acute pain relief in the hospital setting. J Gen Intern Med 2017;32(10):1106–13.

Updates on Multimodal Analgesia for Orthopedic Surgery

Darsi N. Pitchon, MD*, Amir C. Dayan, MD, Eric S. Schwenk, MD,
Jaime L. Baratta, MD, Eugene R. Viscusi, MD

KEYWORDS

- Multimodal analgesia • Orthopedic surgery • Acetaminophen • Ketorolac
- Ibuprofen • Celecoxib • Ketamine • Gabapentinoids

KEY POINTS

- Multimodal analgesia improves analgesic outcomes after orthopedic surgery and minimizes opioids and their side effects.
- Newer nonopioid agents, including IV acetaminophen, IV ibuprofen, and intranasal (IN) ketorolac, are effective multimodal analgesics but cost considerably more than oral formulations and the cost-benefit ratio should be considered when using them.
- Gabapentinoids can help reduce postoperative opioid consumption and improve analgesia after orthopedic surgery.
- Celecoxib can reduce postoperative opioid consumption and improve analgesia after orthopedic surgery.
- Ketamine is a potent analgesic that is most useful in very painful surgery and in opioid-tolerant patients and may be considered for orthopedic surgery.

INTRODUCTION

Orthopedic surgery was one of the first specialties to embrace multimodal analgesia and incorporate it into practice more than a decade ago. Orthopedic surgeries are considered to be some of the most painful procedures patients undergo. Multimodal analgesia, which asserts that the combination of medications with different mechanisms of action provide superior pain relief and fewer side effects compared with a

Disclosure Statement: D.N. Pitchon, A.C. Dayan, and J.L. Baratta have no financial disclosures. E.S. Schwenk has received consulting fees from Avenue Therapeutics. E.R. Viscusi has received research grants from Pacira (080-10000-J19302; 080-10000-J17302) and Durect (080-10000-J13502) and consulting fees from AcelRx, Cara, Egalet, Frezenius, Mallinckrodt, Merck, Heron, Pacira, Pfizer, Salix, and Trevena.
Department of Anesthesiology, Sidney Kimmel Medical College, Thomas Jefferson University, Suite 8290, Gibbon Building, 111 South 11th Street, Philadelphia, PA 19107, USA
* Corresponding author.
E-mail address: Darsi.Pitchon@jefferson.edu

Anesthesiology Clin 36 (2018) 361–373
https://doi.org/10.1016/j.anclin.2018.05.001
1932-2275/18/© 2018 Elsevier Inc. All rights reserved.

anesthesiology.theclinics.com

single class of medication, improves analgesic outcomes in orthopedic surgery.[1] This approach emphasizes using nonopioid adjuncts, such as acetaminophen, nonsteroidal anti-inflammatory drugs (NSAIDs), N-methyl-D-aspartate (NMDA)-receptor antagonists, gabapentinoids, α_2-receptor agonists, and local anesthetics. With the current opioid epidemic in the United States, an emphasis on multimodal analgesia is essential to minimize unnecessary opioid use and manage opioid-tolerant patients. Additionally, multimodal analgesia may help promote early mobilization and discharge, lead to fewer readmission rates, and improve patient satisfaction.[2,3]

To understand the basis for multimodal analgesia, a review of the physiology of pain and its transmission is helpful. The nervous system is made up of a complex system of peripheral nociceptors that extract information from the environment and carry these signals to the central nervous system where they are processed, interpreted, and lead to a physiologic effect. Multiple pain sites may be targeted to disrupt its transmission (**Fig. 1**). At a basic level, pain is divided into nociceptive and neuropathic types. Nociceptive pain occurs with tissue damage, whereas neuropathic pain occurs after damage to the nerve itself. Based on the type, location, and severity of pain experienced by the patient, one or more sites in the pain pathway may be targeted. For example, local anesthetics (via peripheral nerve blocks, neuraxial blocks, intravenous [IV] route, or wound infiltration) provide effective relief for nociceptive (somatic) pain. Neuropathic pain can often be treated with gabapentinoids (gabapentin or pregabalin) or NMDA-receptor antagonists, such as ketamine. Pain after orthopedic surgery is often complex, and it is with this understanding that we describe specific agents used in orthopedic surgery in this article with particular focus on newer agents (**Table 1**).

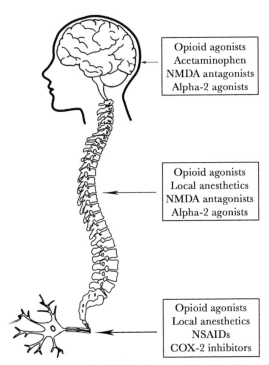

Fig. 1. Multimodal analgesic sites of action in the central and peripheral nervous systems. COX, cyclooxygenase.

Table 1
Multimodal agents commonly used in orthopedic surgery

Drug	Route	Preoperative Dose	Intraoperative Dose	Postoperative Dose
Acetaminophen	IV/PO	1000 mg (>50 kg)	1000 mg	1000 mg q 6 h
Celecoxib	PO	400 mg	N/A	200 mg q 12 h
Gabapentin	PO	800–1200 mg	N/A	300–800 mg q 8 h
Ketamine	IV	N/A	0.5 mg/kg bolus	0.25 mg/kg/h infusion
Ketorolac	IN	31.5 mg	N/A	31.5 mg q 6–8 h
Ibuprofen	IV/PO	600–800 mg	N/A	600 g q 6 h
Pregabalin	PO	75–150 mg	N/A	75 mg q 12 h

Abbreviations: IN, intranasal; IV, intravenous; N/A, not applicable; PO, by mouth.

ACETAMINOPHEN

IV acetaminophen (Ofirmev, Mallinckrodt Pharmaceuticals, St. Louis, MO) was approved for use in the United States by the Food and Drug Administration in 2011.[4] It is speculated that its analgesic mechanism is via activation of descending serotonergic pathways in the central nervous system and via the inhibition of prostaglandin synthesis.[4–7] Some studies link its antinociceptive properties to activation of transient receptor potential vanilloid 1 by a metabolite of acetaminophen, N-arachidonoylphenolamine (AM404), an endogenous cannabinoid.[8,9] In adults and adolescents greater than 50 kg, IV acetaminophen may be dosed 1000 mg every 6 hours or 650 mg every 4 hours up to 4000 mg per day; in patients less than 50 kg, the dose is 15 mg/kg every 6 hours or 12.5 mg/kg every 4 hours to a maximum of 75 mg/kg per day.[5] It has a proven safety record[10] with few contraindications and drug interactions.

In 2005 and 2011, Sinatra and colleagues[11,12] studied the efficacy of IV acetaminophen after total hip arthroplasty and total knee arthroplasty (TKA). In a repeated-dose, randomized, double-blind, placebo-controlled, parallel-group study, 151 patients were given either 1 g IV acetaminophen, IV propacetamol (a prodrug of acetaminophen), or placebo for moderate to severe pain on postoperative day 1. The study group had decreased pain, total opioid consumption, and longer median time to morphine rescue compared with placebo. Patient satisfaction was also improved.

Yang and colleagues[13] performed a meta-analysis to determine the analgesic effect of IV acetaminophen in total joint arthroplasty. Most studies were of low quality; however, there was a significant decrease in pain and opioid consumption on postoperative day 1 to 3. Nausea and vomiting were decreased in acetaminophen groups.

The biggest drawback of IV acetaminophen is the cost. According to one study, 1 g of oral and IV acetaminophen costs $0.03 and $42.25, respectively.[14] Langford and colleagues[15] compared the pharmacokinetics of IV and oral acetaminophen and found that peak plasma concentrations were greater and achieved earlier with the IV formulation. Although they were unable to draw definitive conclusions regarding differences in cerebrospinal fluid concentrations because of small sample size, Singla and colleagues[16] demonstrated faster and greater cerebrospinal fluid penetration with IV versus oral formulations of acetaminophen in a pharmacokinetic study. They demonstrated a 76% higher maximum plasma concentration (C_{max}) and 60% higher maximum cerebrospinal fluid concentration with IV versus oral acetaminophen.[16]

The effectiveness of IV and oral acetaminophen has been compared in studies. O'Neal and colleagues[17] performed a single-center, randomized, double-blind, placebo-controlled trial in 174 patients after TKA under spinal anesthesia comparing IV with oral acetaminophen given at the end of surgery. All patients also received a peri-articular infiltration of ropivacaine, ketorolac, epinephrine, and clonidine. They reported no differences in pain, opioid consumption, and various other pain markers. Of note, the post-anesthesia care unit (PACU) pain ratings and total opioid consumption were low across all groups. Additionally, acetaminophen was only administered once during a time when the spinal still had not worn off, so the peak effect may have been masked. In another randomized prospective trial, 120 patients undergoing hip and knee arthroplasty were given either IV or oral acetaminophen preoperatively and then every 6 hours postoperatively for a total of 24 hours.[18] No differences were found between the two groups except for lower pain ratings during a single time point in the IV group.

In a systematic review of IV versus oral acetaminophen, the authors concluded that for patients who can tolerate oral medications, IV acetaminophen offers no advantage.[19] Given its price in today's cost-conscious health care environment, an assessment of cost versus benefit should occur before use.

INTRANASAL KETOROLAC

Ketorolac is an NSAID with analgesic, antipyretic, and anti-inflammatory properties. It exerts its effects by inhibiting cyclooxygenase (COX) 1 and 2 enzymes, and thus, the synthesis of prostaglandins.[20] When prostaglandins are released at sites of tissue injury, they sensitize nerve terminals leading to a hyperalgesic response. By decreasing the synthesis of prostaglandins, the hyperalgesic response is attenuated and pain is diminished.[21] Intranasal (IN) ketorolac (Sprix, Egalet, Wayne, PA) has the same pharmacokinetic profile, side effect profile, and half-life as an intramuscular injection, with the convenience of IN administration and the potency of morphine.[21,22] It was approved in 2010 for the "short-term treatment of moderate to moderately severe pain for up to 5 days in adult patients who require opioid-strength pain relief."[23] The recommended dose is 31.5 mg (one 15.75-mg spray per nostril) every 6 to 8 hours with a maximum daily dose of 126 mg for a maximum of 5 days.[24]

A phase 3, randomized, double-blind, placebo-controlled trial was performed examining efficacy and tolerability of IN ketorolac in hysterectomy or hip arthroplasty patients.[25] Compared with placebo, 30 mg IN ketorolac provided superior analgesia and lower opioid consumption and decreased constipation and pruritus.

Moodie and colleagues[26] performed a double-blind, randomized, placebo-controlled study comparing the effects of 10 or 30 mg of IN ketorolac with placebo in 127 patients undergoing major abdominal and orthopedic procedures. Patients receiving 30 mg used significantly less morphine compared with the 10-mg and placebo group. The 30-mg IN ketorolac group also demonstrated significantly lower pain ratings, and lower rates of pyrexia and tachycardia.

Pergolizzi and colleagues[27] performed a comprehensive review of IN ketorolac as part of a multimodal approach to postoperative pain. Included in the analysis were the two studies described previously, a large study of 321 patients undergoing major abdominal surgery,[28] and another study including 80 patients undergoing dental surgery.[29] They concluded that the use of IN ketorolac for patients in these four studies led to significantly improved pain intensity at 6 hours and up to 48 hours after surgery.[28]

IN ketorolac is an opioid-sparing analgesic that has demonstrated analgesic properties that are comparable with, or better than, commonly prescribed oral opioids and should be considered in the perioperative period.[30] One drawback, however, is the cost. On GoodRX.com, for example, the price of 5 days of treatment with IN ketorolac is more than $1000.[31]

INTRAVENOUS IBUPROFEN

IV ibuprofen (Caldolor, Cumberland Pharmaceuticals, Nashville, TN) is a nonselective COX inhibitor and acts as an analgesic, antipyretic and anti-inflammatory medication. It was approved by the Food and Drug Administration in 2009 to treat fever and mild to moderate pain or moderate to severe pain as an opioid adjuvant.[32] Recommended dosing for analgesia is 400 mg to 800 mg IV given in a dilute solution over 30 minutes every 6 hours as needed with the highest recommended dose being 2400 mg.[32] Unlike ketorolac, IV ibuprofen does not have a warning on its label about use before major surgery.[33]

In a phase 3, randomized, multicenter, double-blind, placebo-controlled trial, Martinez and colleagues[34] sought to evaluate the safety and efficacy of IV ibuprofen for the treatment of surgical pain in a mixed population with some orthopedic but mostly abdominal surgical patients. They reported a decrease in morphine requirements and pain in the group receiving 800 mg IV ibuprofen every 6 hours compared with placebo for patients undergoing abdominal surgery. No adverse events related to the study drug were noted. IV ibuprofen was efficacious and well tolerated in this mixed population, although the authors were unable to comment on efficacy in the orthopedic population.

In a multicenter, randomized, double-blinded, placebo-controlled study, Singla and colleagues[35] evaluated the safety and efficacy of IV ibuprofen for acute postoperative pain. The study population included patients undergoing elective knee or hip replacement or reconstruction. A dose of 800 mg of IV ibuprofen was administered every 6 hours starting with general anesthesia (GA) induction and continued for 24 hours, followed by every 6 hours as needed for up to 5 days. IV morphine was available via patient-controlled analgesia. During the 6- to 28-hour postoperative period, patients receiving the study drug demonstrated a decrease in pain ratings and morphine consumption when compared with placebo. The use of the study medication dropped dramatically by the 38th hour postsurgery, making any efficacy comparisons for the later time points underpowered. Because bleeding is a concern with the administration of NSAIDs perioperatively, the number of packed red blood cell transfusions and adverse bleeding events were examined and no differences were found between groups. It is worth noting that some high-risk patients receiving full anticoagulation were excluded.

Southworth and colleagues[36] examined the safety and efficacy of IV ibuprofen versus placebo in a multicenter, randomized, double-blind, placebo-controlled trial consisting of adult patients aged 18 to 70 years undergoing orthopedic and major abdominal procedures. The orthopedic procedures consisted of replacement or reconstruction of the knee, hip, or shoulder joints and comprised 111 patients. Although exclusion criteria were extensive, patients receiving 800 mg IV ibuprofen had significantly reduced pain ratings with movement and at rest compared with placebo, whereas patients receiving 400 mg IV ibuprofen showed only a significant difference in pain score with movement. There was a significantly reduced rate of pyrexia in the control groups and an increased incidence of dizziness in the 800-mg IV ibuprofen group. There were no differences in the rates of bleeding or blood transfusions between groups.

In a study examining the pharmacokinetic effects of IV ibuprofen, Smith and Voss[37] demonstrated that although 400 mg of oral ibuprofen maintained 100% bioavailability, faster and greater maximum plasma concentration was achieved with the IV formulation (400 mg and 800 mg). Additionally, the time to maximum plasma concentration was significantly shortened with faster infusion rates (ie, 5–7 minutes as compared with 30- and 60-minute infusions), and the oral formulations never reached the C_{max} achieved by the IV formulations.[37] Head-to-head studies of IV versus oral ibuprofen are lacking, but pharmacologic studies provide some guidance. In the same study, oral ibuprofen reached its peak effect within 90 minutes, whereas IV ibuprofen reached its peak effect anywhere from 10 minutes to 60 minutes depending on the rate of the infusion.[37] Plasma concentrations of ibuprofen were similar about 60 minutes after dosing both the IV and oral formulations, and thus the benefit of the IV formulation in a patient who is able to take oral medications has not been established.[37]

According to RxUSA, the cost of an 800-mg dose of IV ibuprofen is $12.69, whereas the cost of an 800-mg oral ibuprofen tablet is $0.25.[38] Without comparative studies, it is difficult to clearly elucidate a clinical benefit for IV ibuprofen, and further studies are warranted. Additionally, as with other NSAIDs, caution or avoidance should be exercised in patients with asthma, heart failure, bleeding disorders, peptic ulcer disease, inflammatory bowel disease, liver or renal impairment, hyperkalemia, and those who are pregnant, breastfeeding, or younger than 18 years of age. Lower doses and shorter durations of treatment are recommended for patients greater than 65 years because of decreased drug metabolism, decreased cardiac function, and increased risk of gastrointestinal adverse events.[32]

CELECOXIB

Celecoxib (Celebrex, Pfizer, New York, NY) is a selective COX-2 inhibitor indicated for the treatment of pain and inflammation related to osteoarthritis, rheumatoid arthritis, ankylosing spondylitis, acute pain, and primary dysmenorrhea.[39] It carries the same precautions as other NSAIDS, including a black box warning for cardiac thrombotic events, gastrointestinal bleeding, and heart failure, and is contraindicated in the setting of coronary bypass surgery, asthma, or hypersensitivity reactions to NSAIDS or sulfonamides.[40] As a selective COX-2 inhibitor, there is platelet-function sparing and decreased risk for gastrointestinal bleeding compared with nonselective COX inhibitors, but its long-term use has been associated with an increased risk for myocardial infarction and cerebrovascular stroke because of its prothrombotic effects.[41] Rofecoxib (Vioxx, Merck Kenilworth, NJ), approved as a selective COX-2 inhibitor in 1999, was another member of the coxib class, but was later found to have an association with significant cardiovascular events that were underreported in clinical trials. The drug was eventually removed from the market in 2004.[40] Celecoxib may carry a lower risk of cardiovascular events than rofecoxib because it is structurally different and less COX-2-selective. The cardiovascular effects of celecoxib may be related to the duration of use.[42]

Celecoxib is cost-effective at approximately $1 per pill, which may provide up to 24 hours of analgesia.[43] For the management of acute pain, the recommended dose is 400 mg initially, followed by an additional 200-mg dose if needed on the first day. On subsequent days, the dose is 200 mg twice daily as needed.[39]

In a prospective, randomized, placebo-controlled trial of 53 patients undergoing arthroscopic surgery of the hip, Zhang and colleagues[43] compared the effects of 200-mg celecoxib administered 1 hour before surgery with placebo on pain ratings and opioid requirements. There was a significant difference in visual analogue scale (VAS) ratings at the 12- and 24-hour time points in the control group compared with placebo, but no difference in the immediate postoperative recovery period between the two groups. Additionally, patients in the control group had significantly less opioid usage and better Physical Composite Scores at 12 and 24 hours postoperatively, which measured patients' overall physical abilities.

Zhou and colleagues[44] demonstrated decreased VAS ratings and opioid consumption with 400-mg celecoxib administered either 24 hours or 1 hour before surgery compared with placebo in a prospective, randomized, controlled study of 206 patients undergoing arthroscopic knee surgery. Of note, the study was not blinded.

In a prospective, randomized, double-blinded, placebo-controlled study, Kahlenberg and colleagues[45] demonstrated a statistically significant decrease in VAS pain ratings 1 hour after surgery with preoperative administration of 400-mg celecoxib compared with placebo (4.6 vs 5.4) in patients undergoing hip arthroplasty. Although the results were statistically significant, previous studies have quantified a difference of 1.0 to 1.3 on a 10-point VAS scale as clinically significant.[46–49] The control group demonstrated a significant difference in PACU discharge time compared with placebo (152.9 minutes vs 172.9 minutes), which may be more clinically meaningful. There was no difference in opioid consumption between groups.

A systematic review of randomized controlled trials by Shin and colleagues[50] concluded that preoperative oral celecoxib was an effective form of analgesia to decrease postoperative opioid requirements. In patients with no contraindications to celecoxib, it is a safe, efficacious, and cost-effective addition to a multimodal pain regimen when given 1 hour before incision.

GABAPENTINOIDS

Gabapentinoids have gained popularity as part of a multimodal approach to postsurgical pain management. Introduced in the mid-1990s, gabapentin, a synthetic analogue of γ-aminobutyric acid, was initially approved as an anticonvulsant.[51] Since that time, this class of drug has been used for treatment of acute postsurgical pain. The most widely recognized substrate target for gabapentin and pregabalin is the alpha-2 delta-1 subunit of N-type voltage-gated calcium channels, which is upregulated in spinal cord neurons following injury. Binding of these drugs to the alpha-2 delta-1 subunit suppresses the release of neurotransmitters, such as substance P, which subsequently decreases neuronal excitability.[52]

Although specific perioperative doses remain unclear, higher doses of gabapentin (1200 mg) and pregabalin (300 mg) are significantly more effective than lower doses. In addition, the continuation of gabapentin or pregabalin postoperatively is likely more effective than a single preoperative dose.[53]

Several small, randomized controlled trials have demonstrated postoperative benefit of preemptive gabapentinoid use in patients undergoing orthopedic procedures. Montazeri and colleagues[54] randomized 70 healthy patients undergoing lower extremity orthopedic surgery under GA to receive either 300 mg of oral gabapentin or placebo preoperatively. Patients in the gabapentin group had significantly lower VAS ratings at all time intervals up to 24 hours and significantly less morphine consumption in the first 24 hours after surgery. A similar randomized controlled trial performed by Hamal and colleagues[55] examined healthy patients undergoing lower extremity orthopedic surgery under spinal anesthesia. Gabapentin, 600 mg, was given to the treatment group 2 hours before surgery. VAS ratings were reduced at 2 and 24 hours and total opioid consumption in the first 24 hours after surgery was significantly reduced.

A recent triple-blinded, randomized, controlled trial by Mardani-Kivi and colleagues[56] compared 600 mg preoperative oral gabapentin with placebo in patients undergoing shoulder arthroscopy under GA. The pain intensity ratings at 6 hours and 24 hours were not significantly different between treatment and placebo groups. Opioid consumption, however, was significantly reduced in the treatment group at both time points. Nausea and vomiting were also reduced in the treatment group at 6 hours. One meta-analysis concluded that both pain up to 48 hours postoperatively and opioid consumption up to 24 hours postoperatively were reduced in patients undergoing total hip arthroplasty who received gabapentin[57]; similar results have been reported for TKA.[58]

Pregabalin (Lyrica, Pfizer, New York, NY), a newer gabapentinoid, has been less frequently studied. A recent meta-analysis by Dong and colleagues[59] examined the effect of preoperative pregabalin use in TKA. With data from six clinical trials and more than 700 patients, the authors concluded that pregabalin decreased pain and cumulative morphine consumption at 24 and 48 hours after TKA without increasing nausea or vomiting.

The efficacy of gabapentin versus pregabalin for postsurgical pain has not been widely studied. Pregabalin is currently not available in generic form, so it is costlier than gabapentin. Khetarpal and colleagues[60] compared 300 mg pregabalin versus 1200 mg of gabapentin and placebo in patients undergoing lower extremity orthopedic surgery under combined spinal-epidural anesthesia. They concluded that both pregabalin and gabapentin significantly reduced the need for postoperative rescue analgesia, epidural top-offs, and increased the duration of post-spinal anesthesia when compared with placebo. Pregabalin was also found to be superior to gabapentin and placebo at prolonging postoperative pain-free intervals. Of note, pregabalin may potentiate opioid-induced respiratory depression[61] so caution should be taken, particularly in high-risk patients, such as those with obstructive sleep apnea and the elderly. The difference in cost between gabapentin and pregabalin remains significant. A 300-mg capsule of gabapentin is about $0.13,[62] whereas a 75-mg capsule of pregabalin costs about $7.50.[63]

KETAMINE

Ketamine is a dissociative anesthetic, functioning as an antagonist of the NMDA receptor, which provides potent analgesia. At subanesthetic doses, ketamine helps modulate central sensitization and provides antihyperalgesic effects.[64] Animal studies have shown benefit of NMDA antagonists in preventing development of opioid tolerance[65] and reversing opioid-induced tolerance.[66]

Nielsen and colleagues[67] studied 147 surgical spine patients with opioid dependency comparing intraoperative ketamine infusions with placebo. IV patient-controlled analgesia morphine consumption was significantly reduced in the ketamine group, with a mean difference of 42 mg. Similarly, Loftus and colleagues[68] showed significant improvement up to 6 weeks in acute postoperative pain with intraoperative ketamine use for spine patients taking chronic opioids. The authors recommended a 0.5 mg/kg bolus of ketamine followed by an infusion of 0.25 mg/kg/h. Although these recommendations were for opioid-tolerant patients, the dosing suggestions seem appropriate for multimodal therapy based on our experience. Urban and colleagues[69] also reported improved short-term analgesia in opioid-tolerant patients who underwent spine surgery. At least one study, however, by Subramaniam and colleagues[70] did not show significant differences with ketamine use.

Although ketamine in spine surgery has been fairly well studied, a few recent reports have focused on total joint surgery, in particular TKA. Cengiz and colleagues[71] performed a randomized, double-blind, placebo-controlled trial comparing subanesthetic ketamine infusions with saline in 60 patients undergoing TKA under GA. They found that the ketamine group had longer times to first analgesic request postoperatively, reduced morphine consumption, and significantly lower VAS pain ratings. Kadic and colleagues[72] also performed a randomized controlled trial in TKA patients, randomizing patients to receive pregabalin and ketamine or placebo. They noted reduced opioid consumption in the treatment group, but higher rates of adverse effects, such as diplopia and dizziness.

Identifying patients who may benefit from ketamine should be done preoperatively. Involvement of an acute pain service, if available, can help coordinate services and eliminate gaps in care.[73] Routine use of ketamine outside of the operating room has been limited by concerns for psychomimetic effects, including hallucinations, vivid dreams, dissociative feelings, and sedation. Although they may occur at subanesthetic doses, Laskowski and colleagues[74] concluded in their review that no serious events occurred and most adverse effects were mild. This was confirmed in a retrospective review of the use of ketamine on general medical floors, where the authors reported that almost 95% of adverse effects resolved immediately after infusion discontinuation.[75] Still, careful patient selection and caution in the elderly is prudent.

Ketamine is an effective and low-cost perioperative adjuvant. The cost of IV ketamine ranges from $0.38 to $0.59 per milliliter.[76]

SUMMARY

Multimodal analgesia for orthopedic surgery is now widely practiced as a means to reduce opioids and opioid related side effects. A multimodal approach is likely to produce superior analgesia than an opioid-based approach because multimodal analgesic agents target a variety of pain pathways (see **Fig. 1**). Many nonopioid multimodal agents are inexpensive generic drugs. Newer on-patent drugs come at a cost. Practitioners must carefully weigh the value proposition of incorporating these novel drugs. Further work is needed to fully understand this value for many novel agents. In the context of the opioid crisis, a nonopioid, multimodal approach is advisable for all orthopedic procedures whenever possible.

REFERENCES

1. Halawi MJ, Grant SA, Bolognesi MP. Multimodal analgesia for total joint arthroplasty. Orthopedics 2015;38:e616–25.
2. Kohring JM, Orgain NG. Multimodal analgesia in foot and ankle surgery. Orthop Clin North Am 2017;4:495–505.
3. Kehlet H, Wilmore D. Multimodal strategies to improve surgical outcome. Am J Surg 2002;6:630–41.
4. Smith HS. Perioperative intravenous acetaminophen and NSAIDS. Pain Med 2011;12:961–81.
5. Cadence Pharmaceuticals, Inc. 2010. Ofirmev label. Available at: https://www.accessdata.fda.gov/drugsatfda_docs/label/2010/022450lbl.pdf. Accessed November 1, 2017.
6. Graham GG, Scott KF. Mechanism of action paracetamol. Am J Ther 2005;1:46–55.
7. Smith HS. Potential analgesic mechanism of acetaminophen. Pain Physician 2009;12:269–80.
8. Mallet C, Barriere DA, Ermund A, et al. TRPV1 in brain is involved in acetaminophen-induced antinociception. PLoS One 2010;9:1–11.
9. Bertolini A, Ferrari A, Ottani A, et al. Paracetamol: new vistas of an old drug. CNS Drug Rev 2006;3-4:250–75.
10. Candiotti KA, Bergese SD, Viscusi ER, et al. Safety of multiple-dose intravenous acetaminophen in adult inpatients. Pain Med 2010;12:1841–8.

11. Sinatra RS, Jahr JS, Reynolds LW, et al. Efficacy and safety of single and repeated administration of 1 gram intravenous acetaminophen injection (paracetamol) for pain management after major orthopedic surgery. Anesthesiology 2005; 102:822–31.

12. Sinatra RS, Jahr JS, Reynolds LW, et al. Intravenous acetaminophen for pain after major orthopedic surgery: an expanded analysis. Pain Pract 2012;5:357–65.

13. Yang L, Du S, Sun Y. Intravenous acetaminophen as an adjunct to multimodal analgesia after total knee and hip arthroplasty: a systematic review and meta-analysis. Int J Surg 2017;47:135–46.

14. Gallipani A, Mathis SA, Ghin HL, et al. Adverse effect profile comparison of pain regimens with and without intravenous acetaminophen in total hip and knee arthroplasty patients. SAGE Open Med 2017;5:1–7.

15. Langford RA, Hogg M, Bjorksten AR, et al. Comparative plasma and cerebrospinal fluid pharmacokinetics of paracetamol after intravenous and oral administration. Anesth Analg 2016;3:610–5.

16. Singla NK, Parulan C, Samson R, et al. Plasma and cerebrospinal fluid pharmacokinetic parameters after single-dose administration of intravenous, oral, or rectal acetaminophen. Pain Pract 2012;7:523–32.

17. O'Neal JB, Freiberg AA, Yelle MD, et al. Intravenous vs oral acetaminophen as an adjunct to multimodal analgesia after total knee arthroplasty: a prospective, randomized, double-blind clinical trial. J Arthroplasty 2017;32:3029–33.

18. Politi JR, Davis RL II, Matrka AK. Randomized prospective trial comparing the use of intravenous versus oral acetaminophen in total joint arthroplasty. J Arthroplasty 2017;32:1125–7.

19. Jibril F, Sharaby S, Mohamed A, et al. Intravenous versus oral acetaminophen for pain: systematic review of current evidence to support clinical decision-making. Can J Hosp Pharm 2015;3:238–47.

20. Boyer KC, McDonald P, Zoetis T. A novel formulation of ketorolac tomethemine for intranasal administration: preclinical safety evaluation. Int J Toxicol 2010;5: 467–78.

21. Gillis JC, Brogden RN. Ketorolac a reappraisal of its pharmacokinetic properties and therapeutic use in pain management. Drugs 1997;53:139–88.

22. McAleer SD, Majid O, Venables E, et al. Pharmacokinetics and safety of ketorolac following single intranasal and intramuscular administration in healthy volunteers. J Clin Pharmacol 2007;47:13–8.

23. Egalet US Inc. SPRIX: official site for patients. Available at: https://www.sprix.com/patient/. Accessed November 13, 2017.

24. U.S. Food and Drug Administration. Sprix (ketorolac tromethamine) Nasal Spray Drug Approval Package. Available at: https://www.accessdata.fda.gov/drugsatfda_docs/nda/2010/022382Orig1s000LBL.pdf. Accessed January 29, 2018.

25. Brown C, Moodie J, Bisley E, et al. Intranasal ketorolac for postoperative pain: a phase 3, double-blind, randomized study. Pain Med 2009;6:1106–14.

26. Moodie JE, Brown CR, Bisley EJ, et al. The safety and analgesic efficacy of intranasal ketorolac in patients with postoperative pain. Anesth Analg 2008;107: 2025–31.

27. Pergolizzi JV, Taylor R, Raffa RB. Intranasal ketorolac as part of a multimodal approach to postoperative pain. Pain Pract 2015;4:378–88.

28. Singla N, Singla S, Minkowitz HS, et al. Intranasal ketorolac for acute postoperative pain. Curr Med Res Opin 2010;26:1915–23.

29. Grant GM, Mehlisch DR. Intranasal ketorolac for pain secondary to third molar impaction surgery: a randomized, double-blind, placebo-controlled trial. J Oral Maxillofac Surg 2010;68:1025–31.
30. Niebler G, Dayno J. Effect size comparison of ketorolac nasal spray and commonly prescribed oral combination opioids for pain relief after third molar extraction surgery. Postgrad Med 2016;1:12–7.
31. Good Rx, Inc. Sprix. Available at: https://www.goodrx.com/sprix?drug-name=sprix. Accessed January 3, 2018.
32. Alveda Pharmaceuticals Inc. Caldolor product monograph. 2012. Available at http://www.alvedapharma.com/pdf/caldolor_pm.pdf. Accessed December 2, 2017.
33. Ketorolac tromethamine injection package insert. Bedford Laboratories. Available at: https://docs.boehringer-ingelheim.com/Prescribing%20Information/PIs/Ben%20Venue_Bedford%20Labs/55390-481-01%20KRL%2030MG/5539048101. Accessed May 27, 2018.
34. Martinez AG, Rodriquez BE, Roca AP, et al. Intravenous ibuprofen for treatment of post-operative pain: a multicenter, double blind, placebo-controlled, randomized clinical trial. PLoS One 2016;11(5):e0154004.
35. Singla N, Rock A, Pavliv L. A multi-center, randomized, double-blind, placebo-controlled trial of intravenous-ibuprofen (IV-ibuprofen) for treatment of pain in post-operative orthopedic adult patients. Pain Med 2010;11:1284–93.
36. Southworth S, Peters J, Rock A, et al. A multi-center, randomized, double-blind, placebo-controlled trial of intravenous ibuprofen 400 and 800 mg every 6 hours in the management of postoperative pain. Clin Ther 2009;9:1922–35.
37. Smith HS, Voss B. Pharmacokinetics of intravenous ibuprofen: implications of time of infusion in the treatment of pain and fever. Drugs 2012;3:327–37.
38. RxUSA Pharmacy. Ibuprofen. Available at https://rxusa.com/cgi-bin2/db/db.cgi?name2=Ibuprofen. Accessed January 29, 2018.
39. Pfizer, Inc. 2017. Celebrex label. Available at: http://labeling.pfizer.com/showlabeling.aspx?id=793. Accessed December 14, 2017.
40. Krumholz HM, Ross JS, Presler AH, et al. What have we learnt from Vioxx? BMJ 2007;334(7585):120–3.
41. Oviedo JA, Schroy PC III. Does celecoxib use increase the risk of cardiovascular events? Gastroenterology 2005;129(4):1348–50.
42. Fossilien E. Cardiovascular complications of non-steroidal anti-inflammatory drugs. Ann Clin Lab Sci 2005;35:347–85.
43. Zhang Z, Zhu W, Zhu L, et al. Efficacy of celecoxib for pain management after arthroscopic surgery of hip: a prospective randomized placebo-controlled study. Eur J Orthop Surg Traumatol 2014;24:919–23.
44. Zhou F, Du Y, Huang W, et al. The efficacy and safety of early initiation of preoperative analgesia with celecoxib in patients underwent arthroscopic knee surgery. Medicine 2017;96(42):e8234.
45. Kahlenberg CA, Patel RM, Knesek M, et al. Efficacy of celecoxib for early postoperative pain management in hip arthroplasty: a prospective randomized placebo-controlled study. Arthroscopy 2017;6:1180–5.
46. Farrar JT, Young JP Jr, LaMoreaux L, et al. Clinical importance of changes in chronic pain intensity measured on an 11-point numerical pain rating scale. Pain 2001;94:149–58.
47. Hägg O, Fritzell P, Nordwall A, Swedish Lumbar Spine Study Group. The clinical importance of changes in outcome scores after treatment for chronic low back pain. Eur Spine J 2003;12:12–20.

48. Carragee EJ, Cheng I. Minimum acceptable outcomes after lumbar spinal fusion. Spine J 2010;10:313–20.
49. Gallagher EJ, Liebman M, Bijur PE. Prospective validation of clinically important changes in pain severity measured on a visual analog scale. Ann Emerg Med 2001;38:633–8.
50. Shin JJ, McCrum CL, Mauro CS, et al. Systematic review of randomized controlled trials and cohort studies. Am J Sports Med 2017. https://doi.org/10. 1177/0363546517734518.
51. Gabapentin package insert. Pfizer, Inc. Available at: https://www.accessdata.fda. gov/drugsatfda_docs/label/2009/020235s041,020882s028,021129s027lbl.pdf. Accessed May 27, 2018.
52. Sills G. The mechanisms of action of gabapentin and pregabalin. Curr Opin Pharmacol 2006;6:108–13.
53. Schmidt PC, Ruchinelli G, Mackey SC, et al. Perioperative gabapentinoids: choice of agent, dose, timing, and effects on chronic postsurgical pain. Anesthesiology 2013;119:1215–21.
54. Montazeri K, Kashefi P, Honarmand A. Pre-emptive gabapentin significantly reduces postoperative pain and morphine demand following lower extremity orthopaedic surgery. Singapore Med J 2007;48(8):748–51.
55. Hamal PK, Shrestha AB, Shrestha RR. Efficacy of preemptive gabapentin for lower extremity orthopedic surgery under subarachnoid block. JNMA J Nepal Med Assoc 2015;53(200):210–3.
56. Mardani-Kivi M, Karimi Mobarakeh M, Keyhani S, et al. Arthroscopic Bankart surgery: does gabapentin reduce postoperative pain and opioid consumption? A triple-blinded randomized clinical trial. Orthop Traumatol Surg Res 2016;102(5): 549–53.
57. Han C, Li XD, Jiang HQ, et al. The use of gabapentin in the management of postoperative pain after total hip arthroplasty: a meta-analysis of randomized controlled trials. J Orthop Surg Res 2016;11:79.
58. Han C, Li XD, Jiang HQ, et al. The use of gabapentin in the management of postoperative pain after total knee arthroplasty: a PRISMA-compliant meta-analysis of randomized controlled trials. Medicine (Baltimore) 2016;95:e3883.
59. Dong J, Li W, Wang Y. The effect of pregabalin on acute postoperative pain in patients undergoing total knee arthroplasty: a meta-analysis. Int J Surg 2016;34:148–60.
60. Khetarpal R, Kataria AP, Bajaj S, et al. Gabapentin vs pregabalin as a premedication in lower limb orthopaedics surgery under combined spinal epidural technique. Anesth Essays Res 2016;10(2):262–7.
61. Myhre M, Diep LM, Stubhaug A. Pregabalin has analgesic, ventilatory, and cognitive effects in combination with remifentanil. Anesthesiology 2016;124:141–9.
62. Prices and Coupons for Gabapentin. Prices and gabapentin coupons - GoodRx. Available at: https://www.goodrx.com/gabapentin. Accessed January 29, 2018.
63. Prices and Coupons for Pregabalin. Prices and pregabalin coupons - GoodRx. Available at: https://www.goodrx.com/pregabalin. Accessed January 29, 2018.
64. Kock MFD, Lavandhomme PM. The clinical role of NMDA receptor antagonists for the treatment of postoperative pain. Best Pract Res Clin Anaesthesiol 2007;21(1): 85–98.
65. Houghton AK, Parsons CG, Headley MP. Mrz 2/579, a fast kinetic NMDA channel blocker, reduces the development of morphine tolerance in awake rats. Pain 2001;91(3):201–7.
66. Shimoyama N, Shimoyama M, Inturrisi CE, et al. Ketamine attenuates and reverses morphine tolerance in rodents. Anesthesiology 1996;85(6):1357–66.

67. Nielsen RV, Fomsgaard JS, Siegel H, et al. Intraoperative ketamine reduces immediate postoperative opioid consumption after spinal fusion surgery in chronic pain patients with opioid dependency: a randomized, blinded trial. Pain 2017; 158(3):463–70.
68. Loftus RW, Yeager MP, Clark JA, et al. Intraoperative ketamine reduces perioperative opiate consumption in opiate-dependent patients with chronic back pain undergoing back surgery. Pain Med 2010;113:639–46.
69. Urban MK, Deau JTY, Wukovits B, et al. Ketamine as an adjunct to postoperative pain management in opioid tolerant patients after spinal fusions: a prospective randomized trial. HSS J 2007;4(1):62–5.
70. Subramaniam K, Akhouri V, Glazer PA, et al. Intra- and postoperative very low dose intravenous ketamine infusion does not increase pain relief after major spine surgery in patients with preoperative narcotic analgesic intake. Pain Med 2011; 12(8):1276–83.
71. Cengiz P, Gokcinar D, Karabeyoglu I, et al. Intraoperative low-dose ketamine infusion reduces acute postoperative pain following total knee replacement surgery: a prospective, randomized double-blind placebo-controlled trial. J Coll Physicians Surg Pak 2014;24(5):299–303.
72. Kadic L, Haren FV, Wilder-Smith O, et al. The effect of pregabalin and s-ketamine in total knee arthroplasty patients: a randomized trial. J Anaesthesiol Clin Pharmacol 2016;32(4):476–82.
73. Pozek JP, Goldberg SF, Baratta JL, et al. Practical management of the opioid-tolerant patient in the perioperative surgical home. Adv Anesth 2017;35(1): 175–90.
74. Laskowski K, Sirling A, McKay WP. A systematic review of intravenous ketamine for postoperative analgesia. Can J Anaesth 2011;58:911–23.
75. Schwenk ES, Goldberg SF, Patel RD, et al. Adverse drug effects and preoperative medication factors related to perioperative low-dose ketamine infusions. Reg Anesth Pain Med 2016;41(4):482–7.
76. Ketamine Prices, Coupons & Patient Assistance Programs. Drugs.com. Available at: https://www.drugs.com/price-guide/ketamine. Accessed January 29, 2018.

Updates in Enhanced Recovery Pathways for Total Knee Arthroplasty

Lisa Kumar, MD[a], Amanda H. Kumar, MD[b],
Stuart A. Grant, MB ChB[b], Jeff Gadsden, MD, FRCPC, FANZCA[b,*]

KEYWORDS

- Enhanced recovery pathway • Enhanced recovery after surgery
- Total knee arthroplasty • Anesthetic technique

KEY POINTS

- Multidisciplinary team work and coordination is required to develop an enhanced recovery pathway after surgery (ERAS) for patients receiving total knee arthroplasty.
- Not all aspects of other ERAS pathways are applicable in total knee arthroplasty.
- The pathway must be tailored to a specific institution and patient population.
- Looking well ahead of admission until well after discharge provides the biggest opportunity for patient-centric gains.

More than 700,000 primary and revision total knee arthroplasty (TKA) procedures are performed annually in the United States, accounting for more than $10 billion in health related costs.[1] These numbers will continue to grow as obesity and osteoarthritis become more prevalent, and as our population demographics shift to a more aged cohort that is active and desires to maintain their functionality. As such, total joint arthroplasty has become a focus for efforts to develop enhanced recovery after surgery (ERAS) protocols with the aim of improving patient outcomes and reducing health care costs. Originally developed for colorectal surgery, ERAS protocols have now been adopted by a variety of other surgical service lines.

Unlike other surgical procedures, patients undergoing joint replacement typically present with pain and decreased mobility. ERAS pathways for joint replacement focus on reducing pain and accelerating the return to functional recovery, goals that are

Disclosure Statement: J. Gadsden has received consulting fees and research grants from Pacira Pharmaceuticals, Inc, and research grants from Mallinckrodt Pharmaceuticals, Inc.
[a] Regional Anesthesiology and Acute Pain Medicine, Department of Anesthesiology, Duke University Medical Center, 2301 Erwin Road, Durham, NC 27710, USA; [b] Department of Anesthesiology, Duke University Medical Center, 2301 Erwin Road, Durham, NC 27710, USA
* Corresponding author.
E-mail address: Jeff.gadsden@duke.edu

Anesthesiology Clin 36 (2018) 375–386
https://doi.org/10.1016/j.anclin.2018.04.007
1932-2275/18/© 2018 Elsevier Inc. All rights reserved.
anesthesiology.theclinics.com

aligned with the purpose of the surgery itself. As shown with other surgeries, ERAS pathways for TKA have resulted in decreased hospital length of stay (LOS), readmission rates, and health care costs.[2,3] Additionally, standardized clinical pathways have been shown to decrease the incidence of perioperative complications, morbidity, and mortality.[4] This review aims to describe common interventions of an ERAS pathway for TKA patients and to examine the evidence supporting these interventions.

PREOPERATIVE OPTIMIZATION

A key principle of ERAS programs is the identification and optimization of patient-related factors that are known to increase perioperative risk of adverse events. One such patient factor is anemia. Patients with preoperative anemia (defined as hemoglobin <12 g/dL in women and <13 g/dL in men in most studies) appear to be at higher risk for transfusion and postoperative morbidity and mortality.[5,6] In one prospective cohort study of more than 7000 noncardiac, elective surgical patients, preoperative anemia was associated with a twofold increase in the risk of death within the first 14 days, an effect that persisted 90 days after surgery.[5] Another prospective observational database study with more than 5000 patients with total hip arthroplasty and TKA found that preoperative anemia was associated with a fourfold higher rate of transfusion during admission, exposing them to transfusion-related complications, as well as a significantly increased readmission rate within 90 days of surgery.[6] Anemia in this cohort was also associated with increased the risk for a prolonged (>5 days) hospital LOS after adjustment for preoperative patient-related risk factors. Preoperative anemia also has been associated with higher risk of periprosthetic joint infection, with the incidence of infection being up to twice as high in anemic patients in a cohort of 15,000 patients.[7]

When anemia is identified preoperatively (commonly defined as hemoglobin <12 g/dL in women and <13 g/dL in men), hemoglobin should be optimized, and corrected if possible to these minimum concentrations (**Fig. 1**). Given enough lead time (several weeks) this can be done with oral iron therapy alone. Those who cannot tolerate oral iron and those who are scheduled for surgery within 21 days should receive intravenous iron therapy. If indicated (eg, severe anemia or anemia unresponsive to iron therapy), erythropoietin supplementation is periodically used for total joint patients.[8] These therapies require time (typically 3–4 weeks to raise the hemoglobin by 1–2 mg/dL in most patients), highlighting the need for early assessment and implementation of therapy. However, when implemented correctly, these anemia corrective pathways have been shown to decrease allogeneic blood transfusion rates and reduce overall costs.[9,10]

Nutritional status is another patient factor that should be assessed and optimized. Preoperative malnutrition (ie, low albumin and transferrin levels) has been linked with delayed wound healing, increased morbidity, and increased hospital LOS.[11] In a recent retrospective review of 4500 revision TKAs, patients with low serum albumin (<3.5 mg/dL) were more likely to develop deep surgical site infections, pneumonia, sepsis, and major perioperative complications, such as unplanned intubation, transfusion, and acute kidney injury.[12] Preoperative nutrition screening tools can be used to assess body mass index, recent weight loss, recent reduction in oral intake, and low serum albumin.[13] If the patient is at high risk, from a nutritional standpoint, a nutrition consult is recommended and a least 7 days of oral nutrition supplementation should be provided.

Cigarette smoking is another known risk factor for poor outcomes, including increased rates of infection, inadequate pain control, pulmonary complications,

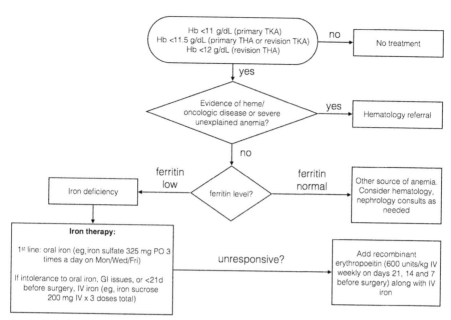

Fig. 1. Sample preoperative anemia treatment pathway. Patients presenting with anemia should undergo evaluation and be considered for iron/erythropoietin supplementation. Hb, hemoglobin; IV, intravenous; PO, oral; THA, total hip arthroplasty.

increased rates of pseudoarthrosis, and poor bone healing.[14] Cessation of smoking 4 weeks before surgery appears to lower risk to approximately the level of non-smokers.[14] Smoking cessation counseling at the time of preoperative assessment can be a relatively simple, low-cost intervention and has been shown to lead to a high proportion (>60%) of patients remaining smoke-free.[15]

SETTING PATIENT EXPECTATIONS

Managing patient expectations of pain, surgical experience, and recovery is critical to achieving high patient satisfaction. Preoperative educational "joint classes" taught by a multidisciplinary team of nurses, case managers, physical therapists, and occupational therapists serve to prepare arthroplasty patients and their families to better handle the events before and after surgery. These classes are designed to address not only physical but also psychosocial issues related to joint replacement. Such classes increase patient engagement in their care, facilitate development of coping strategies, and build patient confidence in their ability to recover from surgery.[16] Discharge disposition (ie, to home or to a rehabilitation or skilled nursing facility) is greatly influenced by patient expectations.[17] Studies that compare live classes versus Web-based or video-taped classes are lacking, although various formats have been used with success.[18] Although patient anxiety and disposition have been shown to be reduced after preoperative education, such classes have not been found to consistently decrease LOS, pain scores, ambulation distances, or complication rates.[19]

Patients with a history of chronic pain can benefit from meeting with an acute pain physician preoperatively, both to set expectations for postsurgical pain ("pain prehabilitation") and to wean preoperative opioids before surgery.[20] Patients who are coached to set realistic pain goals of approximately 3 to 4 of 10 on the Numeric Rating

Scale are less likely to be dissatisfied with their postoperative pain control.[21] Similarly, patients with a history of psychiatric comorbidity, such as anxiety, or those who tend to engage in pain catastrophizing also may benefit from preoperative cognitive-behavioral therapy focused on pain-coping skills.[22] Pain catastrophizing is a behavior pattern in which individuals ruminate about and magnify their pain, and feel helpless to manage their pain.[23] The Pain Catastrophizing Scale is a validated instrument that was developed to quantify this tendency. Individuals scoring high on the scale have a higher chance of developing chronic pain after surgery, although preemptive intervention and counseling may reduce this risk.

Patients on chronic opioid therapy before arthroplasty experience higher in-hospital opioid use, a higher pain intensity, and an increased risk of complications compared with opioid-naïve patients.[24,25] This may be due to both opioid tolerance with consequent undertreatment of the acute pain, as well as the presence of opioid-induced hyperalgesia, a neuropharmacological state in which patients receiving opioids for pain may in fact become more sensitive to pain stimuli.[26] Nguyen and colleagues[27] reported that arthroplasty patients who underwent an opioid-weaning protocol (defined as a ≥50% reduction in opioid dose) performed significantly better on specific measures of health outcomes (University of California, Los Angeles activity score and the Western Ontario and McMaster Universities Arthritis Index) than those who did not participate in the protocol, while performing similar to those patients who were opioid naïve. The implementation of a multidisciplinary, preoperative transitional pain service to identify patients at risk for chronic persistent postoperative pain, and to appropriately tailor a weaning program appears to be both feasible and practical.[28] Moreover, a survey of surgeons from a variety of specialties identified opioid use as one of the chief preoperative modifiable risk factors that should be optimized preoperatively, second only to tobacco use.[29] Screening for patients at risk for chronic pain should continue into the perioperative period.[21,30] Patients with higher pain score trajectories on postoperative days (PODs) 1 through 8 appear to be at risk for worse pain 3 months postoperatively, and may benefit from early identification and aggressive secondary prevention strategies.[31]

PREOPERATIVE PHYSICAL THERAPY AND EXERCISE

Preoperative aerobic exercise regimens, also termed prehabilitation, can decrease morbidity and mortality in certain surgical populations by improving preoperative functional status.[32] Data are limited in TKA patients and, to date, studies have not demonstrated significant benefits in terms of pain scores, functional recovery, hospital LOS, or hospital costs.[33,34] The reason for this may be that patients with osteoarthritis severe enough to warrant surgery are unable to reach the exercise intensity needed to show benefits. Additionally, many of the studies performed on prehabilitation in TKA included only healthy, fit patients; more likely it is the sicker patients who would benefit from a preoperative strengthening and improvement of functional status.[35] Regardless, more studies are needed to determine the utility of prehabilitation for TKA.

TYPE OF SURGICAL ANESTHETIC

The choice of anesthetic technique for TKA depends on several factors, including anticoagulation status, preoperative cardiopulmonary health, patient preferences, and institutional workflow factors, among others. There is a lack of consensus among the anesthesia community as to the superiority of neuraxial versus general anesthesia, as older data have tended to be conflicting.[36,37] However, more recent data, particularly from analyses of large patient databases, may suggest that the pendulum is swinging toward an advantage for spinal anesthesia. Memtsoudis and colleagues[38] performed an analysis of more than 380,000 total knee and hip arthroplasty procedures and demonstrated that general anesthesia was associated with an almost twofold increase in 30-day mortality. Basques and colleagues[39] performed a similar study using the American College of Surgeons NSQIP database and found that general anesthesia was associated with a 25% increase in adverse events compared with spinal anesthesia in this population. Other large database studies performed in the past several years support the favorable effect spinal anesthesia has on morbidity, mortality, and LOS.[40,41] It is worth noting, however, that most of these studies did not specify general anesthetic technique (ie, total intravenous anesthesia vs inhaled volatile anesthetic), the type of airway devices (ie, supraglottic vs endotracheal tubes) or the adjunctive use of peripheral nerve blocks, all factors that may play a role in the recovery profile following arthroplasty. In contrast, when a general anesthetic using target-controlled propofol and remifentanil was compared with spinal anesthesia in prospective study, patients in the general anesthesia group experienced shorter LOS; less nausea, vomiting, and dizziness; and earlier ambulation, suggesting that not all general anesthetics are created equal, and careful attention to enhanced recovery and fast-track principles can reduce some of the differences traditionally seen between anesthetic techniques.[42]

MULTIMODAL ANALGESIC AGENTS

There are many nonopioid medications that can be used as adjuncts for analgesia with the goal of decreasing or eliminating opioid requirements and associated adverse effects. It is well established that analgesia is improved and side effects are reduced when nonopioid analgesics are combined with opioids, and the reduction and/or elimination of opioids is one of the central themes of most contemporary ERAS protocols.[43] It is critically important to establish the nonopioid multimodal agents as scheduled, around-the-clock building blocks of the analgesic plan, and only after that has been established should opioids be prescribed as needed for breakthrough pain.

Nonsteroidal anti-inflammatory drugs (NSAIDs) are widely used for analgesia as well as to reduce inflammation, and should be a foundational element of the ERAS pathway for TKA. Nonselective NSAIDs (eg, ibuprofen, ketorolac) can be associated with gastrointestinal (GI) ulceration and renal side effects if taken for prolonged periods of time and/or in high doses. However, in individuals who tolerate these drugs preoperatively without issue, the benefit of a short (10–14 day) course outweighs this relatively rare risk. Use of cyclooxygenase-2 inhibitors can help to mitigate the GI side effects of nonselective NSAIDs but still have an effect on renal perfusion. Use of celecoxib in the perioperative period results in decreased opioid consumption and improved postoperative range of motion in joint replacement surgery.[44]

Acetaminophen is another commonly used nonopioid, and its combination with NSAIDs provides superior analgesia compared with either drug alone.[45] Acetaminophen also enjoys a relatively favorable side-effect profile. Within the doses used in typical ERAS protocols (1000 mg every 6 hours), there is little concern for hepatic toxicity. Gabapentinoids (eg, gabapentin, pregabalin) act at the voltage-gated calcium channels, and in addition to reducing opioid requirements in the acute recovery period, these agents have been shown to decrease the incidence of chronic pain after TKA.[46] Gabapentinoids are associated with sedation and dizziness, and care must be taken to dose these agents appropriately. It is often prudent to start on the low end of the dosing range (eg, 100 mg orally) and titrate up as tolerated to 300 mg orally every

8 hours. Some institutions favor a single nighttime dose of gabapentin to leverage the sedative effect for patient comfort and satisfaction.

Intraoperative use of subanesthetic, low-dose ketamine has potent analgesic efficacy with limited adverse effects and can be an important adjunct to opioids and other nonopioid analgesics. Ketamine is effective if administered as a single bolus at the time of incision, as it reduces postoperative morphine use in total joint replacement by 25% to 40%.[47] Low-dose ketamine infusion also may reduce the incidence of chronic pain, especially in those patients who present with high opioid use preoperatively, and in particular has been shown to significantly attenuate opioid-induced hyperalgesia in some patients.[48,49]

Dexamethasone is a corticosteroid that is routinely used for prophylaxis against nausea and vomiting. A potent anti-inflammatory, dexamethasone modulates inflammation-related pain pathways and has been used successfully as an analgesic for a variety of surgical procedures in higher doses (>0.1 mg/kg).[50] A recent randomized clinical trial demonstrated that a 10-mg intravenous dose of dexamethasone intraoperatively reduced hospital LOS by an entire day (3.0 vs 3.97 days, $P<.001$).[51] This effect is even more pronounced if the dose is repeated on the first postoperative day.[51] There appear to be no adverse effects of 1 to 2 doses of perioperative dexamethasone on wound healing or infection. However, hyperglycemia may occur in poorly controlled diabetics, and the resulting challenge of having to manage an elevated blood glucose (which *has* been associated with periprosthetic wound infection[52]) compared with potential benefits in this population is unclear.

PERIPHERAL NERVE BLOCKS AND INFILTRATION

Nerve blocks for TKA must balance the need for quality analgesia with the ability to safely stand, pivot, and ambulate. For this reason, adductor canal blocks have largely replaced femoral nerve blocks in practices that offer peripheral nerve blocks, as they provide a sensory block of the anteromedial knee while preserving quadriceps muscle strength, enabling early ambulation after surgery.[53,54] Another source of postoperative pain is the posterior knee, which is innervated by the popliteal plexus, a fine mesh of nerves that arise from the tibial nerve (**Fig. 2**). Much like the femoral nerve block, many centers have moved away from performing sciatic blocks for TKA because of the resulting complete sensorimotor blockade of the calf, foot, and ankle and associated difficulty with ambulation. However, the ultrasound-guided iPACK block (Interspace between the Popliteal Artery and Capsule of the Knee) is a potential solution that appears to provide good posterior knee analgesia while sparing the motor fibers. With this technique, the anesthesiologist obtains a view of the posterior femur and the popliteal vessels just above the knee joint line. A needle is advanced from lateral to medial, and 20 mL of dilute local anesthetic are then deposited between the popliteal artery and the metaphysis of the femur under ultrasound guidance. The popliteal plexus is not seen in this technique, but proper deposition of the local anesthetic just adjacent to the posterior knee capsule results in good posterior pain relief for approximately 18 to 24 hours (when 0.2% ropivacaine is used). Compared with patients who received a femoral catheter alone, patients who also received an iPACK block had significantly decreased postoperative opioid requirements.[55] The iPACK is performed as a single injection, whereas a continuous peripheral nerve catheter can be left in place for the adductor canal block to prolong its analgesic benefits.[56]

Many centers have adopted surgeon-administered local anesthetic infiltration (LIA) of the periarticular soft tissues, a technique that is typically performed with large volumes (approximately 200 mL) of dilute local anesthetic with or without adjuvants such

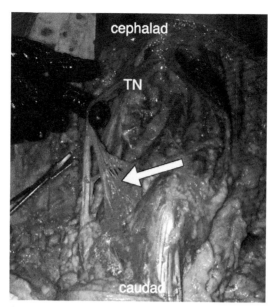

Fig. 2. The popliteal plexus in a cadaver dissection. The web-like plexus (*arrow*) is seen coming off the tibial nerve (TN) before supplying the posterior capsule and soft tissues of the knee joint.

as epinephrine and ketorolac. Some surgeons also choose to also admix opioids and/or steroids into this joint "cocktail." Due to its relative simplicity, it has enjoyed a widespread acceptance, although the data on the efficacy of LIA are somewhat mixed. There appear to be some technique-dependent factors, and infiltration can be performed precisely, with good adherence to anatomic principles, just as it can be performed in a haphazard manner. Those surgeons who appear to take the greatest care with LIA technique report pain, opioid-sparing, and mobility outcomes that are equivalent to nerve block techniques.[57]

REHABILITATION

Postoperative physical therapy beginning on the day of surgery has been shown to decrease hospital LOS. In one study, 147 patients underwent a fast-track rehabilitation program involving mobilization on POD 0, group therapy, and 1:1 physiotherapy for 2 hours daily, and experienced improved joint range of motion, decreased analgesic use, and decreased hospital LOS compared with controls.[58] Another study showed similar results with physical therapy starting 2 to 4 hours after surgery on POD 0. Therapy consisted of bed transfers, moving from a sitting to standing position, and ambulation for 15 to 30 feet with staff assistance.[59] Patients also performed ankle pumping, static quadriceps, and buttock strengthening exercises. Hospital LOS in this study was 69 hours shorter than controls, and patients who received early physiotherapy reported lower pain scores both at rest and with activity, and used decreased morphine equivalents.

FUTURE DIRECTIONS

As we move further along the path of enhanced recovery, our goals will naturally shift and evolve. Whereas not very long ago it was expected to have a TKA patient lying in bed with an epidural and a continuous passive motion machine after surgery, we are now mobilizing these patients at the earliest possible juncture, sometimes while still in the recovery room. It is not unrealistic to predict that the vast majority of TKAs will be performed on an outpatient basis sometime in the next 5 to 7 years. To achieve that, we will need to overcome some of the barriers that continue to keep some patients in hospital. There will always be a cohort that is simply not well enough to be safely discharged home or to a hotel room on the same day. However, unlike colorectal surgical patients who struggle with gut motility, tolerating a diet, and substantial perturbations of fluid homeostasis as their reason for their postoperative hospital stay, for TKA patients the limiting factor is primarily pain and its effects on mobility. As such, future developments that move the needle for orthopedic ERAS protocols will likely have to include the use of new long-acting analgesia techniques that are placed preoperatively, and that can provide prolonged postoperative analgesia. This may include long-acting local anesthetics available now or under development. Preoperative ablation of genicular nerve branches through the use of cryotherapy or radiofrequency ablation is an evolving idea that has garnered much interest.[60,61] If the sensory (but not motor) nerves that supply the knee are "burned away" in a fashion that lasts for several months, this may be as close to an ideal solution as we can imagine. The knee remains a complex joint with nerve supply from at least 3 major branches of the lumbosacral plexus, and it remains to be seen if genicular branches alone could provide significant pain relief.

SUMMARY

ERAS for TKA is an exciting and evolving science. Certainly, what is best practice for knee arthroplasty in 2018 is likely to change by 2023. A continued focus on motor-sparing analgesic techniques, and the elimination (or near elimination) of opioids will be at the heart of these clinical pathways. As the individual patient's experience improves, the other components of the Institute for Healthcare Improvement's Triple Aim (namely, improvements in population health and reduction in costs) may naturally fall in line. As always, there is a need for high-quality data so that the ERAS pathways can be established and continually improved based on evidence.

REFERENCES

1. Kurtz SM, Ong KL, Lau E, et al. International survey of primary and revision total knee replacement. Int Orthop 2011;35(12):1783–9.
2. Macario A, Horne M, Goodman S, et al. The effect of a perioperative clinical pathway for knee replacement surgery on hospital costs. Anesth Analg 1998; 86(5):978–84.
3. Larsen K, Hvass KE, Hansen TB, et al. Effectiveness of accelerated perioperative care and rehabilitation intervention compared to current intervention after hip and knee arthroplasty. A before-after trial of 247 patients with a 3-month follow-up. BMC Musculoskelet Disord 2008;9:59.
4. Malviya A, Martin K, Harper I, et al. Enhanced recovery program for hip and knee replacement reduces death rate. Acta Orthop 2011;82(5):577–81.
5. Beattie WS, Karkouti K, Wijeysundera DN, et al. Risk associated with preoperative anemia in noncardiac surgery: a single-center cohort study. Anesthesiology 2009;110(3):574–81.
6. Jans O, Jorgensen C, Kehlet H, et al, Lundbeck Foundation Centre for Fast-track Hip and Knee Replacement Collaborative Group. Role of preoperative anemia for

risk of transfusion and postoperative morbidity in fast-track hip and knee arthroplasty. Transfusion 2014;54(3):717–26.

7. Greenky M, Gandhi K, Pulido L, et al. Preoperative anemia in total joint arthroplasty: is it associated with periprosthetic joint infection? Clin Orthop Relat Res 2012;470(10):2695–701.

8. Basora M, Colomina MJ, Tio M, et al. Optimizing preoperative haemoglobin in major orthopaedic surgery using intravenous iron with or without erythropoietin. An epidemiologic study. Rev Esp Anestesiol Reanim 2015;62(6):313–21.

9. Guinn NR, Guercio JR, Hopkins TJ, et al. How do we develop and implement a preoperative anemia clinic designed to improve perioperative outcomes and reduce cost? Transfusion 2016;56(2):297–303.

10. Petis SM, Lanting BA, Vasarhelyi EM, et al. Is there a role for preoperative iron supplementation in patients preparing for a total hip or total knee arthroplasty? J Arthroplasty 2017;32(9):2688–93.

11. Berend KR, Lombardi AV Jr, Mallory TH. Rapid recovery protocol for perioperative care of total hip and total knee arthroplasty patients. Surg Technol Int 2004;13:239–47.

12. Kamath AF, Nelson CL, Elkassabany N, et al. Low albumin is a risk factor for complications after revision total knee arthroplasty. J Knee Surg 2017;30(3):269–75.

13. Wischmeyer PE, Carli F, Evans DC, et al. American Society for Enhanced Recovery and Perioperative Quality Initiative joint consensus statement on nutrition screening and therapy within a surgical enhanced recovery pathway. Anesth Analg 2018;126:1883–95.

14. Truntzer J, Vopat B, Feldstein M, et al. Smoking cessation and bone healing: optimal cessation timing. Eur J Orthop Surg Traumatol 2015;25(2):211–5.

15. Akhavan S, Nguyen LC, Chan V, et al. Impact of smoking cessation counseling prior to total joint arthroplasty. Orthopedics 2017;40(2):e323–8.

16. Lane-Carlson ML, Kumar J. Engaging patients in managing their health care: patient perceptions of the effect of a total joint replacement presurgical class. Perm J 2012;16(3):42–7.

17. Halawi MJ, Vovos TJ, Green CL, et al. Patient expectation is the most important predictor of discharge destination after primary total joint arthroplasty. J Arthroplasty 2015;30(4):539–42.

18. Ibrahim MS, Alazzawi S, Nizam I, et al. An evidence-based review of enhanced recovery interventions in knee replacement surgery. Ann R Coll Surg Engl 2013;95(6):386–9.

19. Kearney M, Jennrich MK, Lyons S, et al. Effects of preoperative education on patient outcomes after joint replacement surgery. Orthop Nurs 2011;30(6):391–6.

20. Gadsden J. Enhanced recovery for orthopedic surgery. Int Anesthesiol Clin 2017; 55(4):116–34.

21. Forsythe ME, Dunbar MJ, Hennigar AW, et al. Prospective relation between catastrophizing and residual pain following knee arthroplasty: two-year follow-up. Pain Res Manag 2008;13(4):335–41.

22. Riddle DL, Keefe FJ, Nay WT, et al. Pain coping skills training for patients with elevated pain catastrophizing who are scheduled for knee arthroplasty: a quasi-experimental study. Arch Phys Med Rehabil 2011;92(6):859–65.

23. Osman A, Barrios FX, Kopper BA, et al. Factor structure, reliability, and validity of the pain catastrophizing scale. J Behav Med 1997;20(6):589–605.

24. Chapman CR, Davis J, Donaldson GW, et al. Postoperative pain trajectories in chronic pain patients undergoing surgery: the effects of chronic opioid pharmacotherapy on acute pain. J Pain 2011;12(12):1240–6.

25. Zywiel MG, Stroh DA, Lee SY, et al. Chronic opioid use prior to total knee arthroplasty. J Bone Joint Surg Am 2011;93(21):1988–93.

26. Chu LF, Angst MS, Clark D. Opioid-induced hyperalgesia in humans: molecular mechanisms and clinical considerations. Clin J Pain 2008;24(6):479–96.

27. Nguyen LC, Sing DC, Bozic KJ. Preoperative reduction of opioid use before total joint arthroplasty. J Arthroplasty 2016;31(9 Suppl):282–7.

28. Katz J, Weinrib A, Fashler SR, et al. The Toronto General Hospital Transitional Pain Service: development and implementation of a multidisciplinary program to prevent chronic postsurgical pain. J Pain Res 2015;8:695–702.

29. McAnally H. Rationale for and approach to preoperative opioid weaning: a preoperative optimization protocol. Perioper Med (Lond) 2017;6:19.

30. Burns LC, Ritvo SE, Ferguson MK, et al. Pain catastrophizing as a risk factor for chronic pain after total knee arthroplasty: a systematic review. J Pain Res 2015;8: 21–32.

31. Lavand'homme PM, Grosu I, France MN, et al. Pain trajectories identify patients at risk of persistent pain after knee arthroplasty: an observational study. Clin Orthop Relat Res 2014;472(5):1409–15.

32. Santa Mina D, Scheede-Bergdahl C, Gillis C, et al. Optimization of surgical outcomes with prehabilitation. Appl Physiol Nutr Metab 2015;40(9):966–9.

33. D'Lima DD, Colwell CW Jr, Morris BA, et al. The effect of preoperative exercise on total knee replacement outcomes. Clin Orthop Relat Res 1996;(326):174–82.

34. Hoogeboom TJ, Oosting E, Vriezekolk JE, et al. Therapeutic validity and effectiveness of preoperative exercise on functional recovery after joint replacement: a systematic review and meta-analysis. PLoS One 2012;7(5):e38031.

35. Hoogeboom TJ, Dronkers JJ, Hulzebos EH, et al. Merits of exercise therapy before and after major surgery. Curr Opin Anaesthesiol 2014;27(2):161–6.

36. Rodgers A, Walker N, Schug S, et al. Reduction of postoperative mortality and morbidity with epidural or spinal anaesthesia: results from overview of randomised trials. BMJ 2000;321(7275):1493.

37. Macfarlane AJ, Prasad GA, Chan VW, et al. Does regional anesthesia improve outcome after total knee arthroplasty? Clin Orthop Relat Res 2009;467(9): 2379–402.

38. Memtsoudis SG, Rasul R, Suzuki S, et al. Does the impact of the type of anesthesia on outcomes differ by patient age and comorbidity burden? Reg Anesth Pain Med 2014;39(2):112–9.

39. Basques BA, Toy JO, Bohl DD, et al. General compared with spinal anesthesia for total hip arthroplasty. J Bone Joint Surg Am 2015;97(6):455–61.

40. Perlas A, Chan VW, Beattie S. Anesthesia technique and mortality after total hip or knee arthroplasty: a retrospective, propensity score-matched cohort study. Anesthesiology 2016;125(4):724–31.

41. Saied NN, Helwani MA, Weavind LM, et al. Effect of anaesthesia type on postoperative mortality and morbidities: a matched analysis of the NSQIP database. Br J Anaesth 2017;118(1):105–11.

42. Harsten A, Kehlet H, Toksvig-Larsen S. Recovery after total intravenous general anaesthesia or spinal anaesthesia for total knee arthroplasty: a randomized trial. Br J Anaesth 2013;111(3):391–9.

43. Joshi GP, Schug SA, Kehlet H. Procedure-specific pain management and outcome strategies. Best Pract Res Clin Anaesthesiol 2014;28(2):191–201.

44. Buvanendran A, Kroin JS, Tuman KJ, et al. Effects of perioperative administration of a selective cyclooxygenase 2 inhibitor on pain management and recovery of

function after knee replacement: a randomized controlled trial. JAMA 2003; 290(18):2411–8.

45. Ong CK, Seymour RA, Lirk P, et al. Combining paracetamol (acetaminophen) with nonsteroidal antiinflammatory drugs: a qualitative systematic review of analgesic efficacy for acute postoperative pain. Anesth Analg 2010;110(4):1170–9.

46. Buvanendran A, Kroin JS, Della Valle CJ, et al. Perioperative oral pregabalin reduces chronic pain after total knee arthroplasty: a prospective, randomized, controlled trial. Anesth Analg 2010;110(1):199–207.

47. Elia N, Tramer MR. Ketamine and postoperative pain–a quantitative systematic review of randomised trials. Pain 2005;113(1–2):61–70.

48. Remerand F, Le Tendre C, Baud A, et al. The early and delayed analgesic effects of ketamine after total hip arthroplasty: a prospective, randomized, controlled, double-blind study. Anesth Analg 2009;109(6):1963–71.

49. Choi E, Lee H, Park HS, et al. Effect of intraoperative infusion of ketamine on remifentanil-induced hyperalgesia. Korean J Anesthesiol 2015;68(5):476–80.

50. De Oliveira GS Jr, Almeida MD, Benzon HT, et al. Perioperative single dose systemic dexamethasone for postoperative pain: a meta-analysis of randomized controlled trials. Anesthesiology 2011;115(3):575–88.

51. Backes JR, Bentley JC, Politi JR, et al. Dexamethasone reduces length of hospitalization and improves postoperative pain and nausea after total joint arthroplasty: a prospective, randomized controlled trial. J Arthroplasty 2013;28(8 Suppl):11–7.

52. Yang L, Sun Y, Li G, et al. Is hemoglobin A1c and perioperative hyperglycemia predictive of periprosthetic joint infection following total joint arthroplasty? A systematic review and meta-analysis. Medicine (Baltimore) 2017;96(51): e8805.

53. Jaeger P, Zaric D, Fomsgaard JS, et al. Adductor canal block versus femoral nerve block for analgesia after total knee arthroplasty: a randomized, double-blind study. Reg Anesth Pain Med 2013;38(6):526–32.

54. Kwofie MK, Shastri UD, Gadsden JC, et al. The effects of ultrasound-guided adductor canal block versus femoral nerve block on quadriceps strength and fall risk: a blinded, randomized trial of volunteers. Reg Anesth Pain Med 2013; 38(4):321–5.

55. Thobhani S, Scalercio L, Elliott CE, et al. Novel regional techniques for total knee arthroplasty promote reduced hospital length of stay: an analysis of 106 patients. Ochsner J 2017;17(3):233–8.

56. Ilfeld BM. Continuous peripheral nerve blocks: a review of the published evidence. Anesth Analg 2011;113(4):904–25.

57. Mont MA, Beaver WB, Dysart SH, et al. Local infiltration analgesia with liposomal bupivacaine improves pain scores and reduces opioid use after total knee arthroplasty: results of a randomized controlled trial. J Arthroplasty 2018;33(1): 90–6.

58. den Hertog A, Gliesche K, Timm J, et al. Pathway-controlled fast-track rehabilitation after total knee arthroplasty: a randomized prospective clinical study evaluating the recovery pattern, drug consumption, and length of stay. Arch Orthop Trauma Surg 2012;132(8):1153–63.

59. Raphael M, Jaeger M, van Vlymen J. Easily adoptable total joint arthroplasty program allows discharge home in two days. Can J Anaesth 2011;58(10): 902–10.

60. Ilfeld BM, Gabriel RA, Trescot AM. Ultrasound-guided percutaneous cryoneurolysis for treatment of acute pain: could cryoanalgesia replace continuous peripheral nerve blocks? Br J Anaesth 2017;119(4):703–6.

61. Asenjo A, Arboleda M, Michelagnoli G, et al. Functional outcome and postoperative analgesia following total knee arthoplasty: randomized double-blind comparison between continuous adductor canal block and preoperative radiofrequency ablation of saphenous and genicular nerves. Abstract presented at the 16th Annual ASRA Pain Medicine Meeting. Lake Buena Vista, (FL), November 16, 2017.

Novel Methodologies in Regional Anesthesia for Knee Arthroplasty

Rodney A. Gabriel, MD, MAS (Clinical Research),
Brian M. Ilfeld, MD, MS (Clinical Investigation)*

KEYWORDS

- Knee arthroplasty • Cryoanalgesia • Cryoneurolysis • Neuromodulation
- Peripheral nerve stimulation

KEY POINTS

- Combined with the rising expertise of ultrasound imaging among anesthesiologists, ubiquitous availability of ultrasound devices, and availability of portable cryodevices, cryoanalgesia is now a realistic intervention for acute pain management.
- Although a single application of ultrasound-guided percutaneous cryoneurolysis provides weeks to months of analgesia, careful selection of candidates is required given the potential prolonged motor block if mixed motor-sensory nerves are targeted.
- Ultrasound-guided percutaneous peripheral nerve stimulation offers a novel intervention to provide post–knee arthroplasty analgesia without the major limitations of opioids and continuous peripheral nerve blockade.
- Before ultrasound-guided percutaneous cryoanalgesia and percutaneous peripheral nerve stimulation may be routinely practiced, robust clinical trials documenting their risks and benefits in managing acute and subacute postoperative pain should be conducted.

Disclosures: R.A. Gabriel's institution has received funding and product for his research from Myoscience and Epimed; infusion pump manufacturer Infutronics; perineural catheter manufacturer Ferrosan Medical; and a manufacturer of a peripheral nerve stimulation device, SPR Therapeutics. B.M. Ilfeld's institution has received funding and product for his research from Myoscience and Epimed; infusion pump manufacturer Infutronics; perineural catheter manufacturer Ferrosan Medical; a manufacturer of a peripheral nerve stimulation device, SPR Therapeutics; and, manufacturers of long-acting bupivacaine formulations, Pacira Pharmaceuticals and Heron Pharmaceuticals.
Department of Anesthesiology, University of California, San Diego, 200 West Arbor Drive, MC 8770, San Diego, CA 92103, USA
* Corresponding author.
E-mail address: bilfeld@ucsd.edu

Anesthesiology Clin 36 (2018) 387–401
https://doi.org/10.1016/j.anclin.2018.05.002
1932-2275/18/Published by Elsevier Inc.

anesthesiology.theclinics.com

INTRODUCTION

Maximizing analgesia is critical following joint arthroplasty because postoperative pain is a major barrier to adequate participation in physical therapy, which is in itself central to optimizing functional recovery. Both single-injection and continuous peripheral nerve blocks (PNB) provide pain control following knee arthroplasty[1] and are often considered the gold standard for postoperative analgesia.[2] However, limitations of these techniques have limited their general use,[3,4] and alternatives could improve the risk-benefit ratio and increase their application worldwide following knee arthroplasty.

One of the major issues of local anesthetic-based analgesics is their duration measured in only a few hours or days. The pain following total knee arthroplasty (TKA) usually far outlasts this analgesic duration. The duration of continuous PNB catheters is limited by the risk of infection and dislodgement.[5] Perineural infusions also induce motor, sensory, and proprioception deficits that potentially increase the risk of falling.[4] A further disadvantage of continuous PNB in ambulatory patients is the burden of carrying an infusion pump and local anesthetic reservoir bag. Percutaneous cryoneurolysis and peripheral nerve stimulation (PNS) are two modalities approved by the Food and Drug Administration (FDA) for use in treating acute pain; yet they have been nearly absent from the acute pain literature.[6–8] This article reviews these analgesic methods and their application to acute pain states, specifically for knee arthroplasty.

CRYOANALGESIA

Cryoanalgesia, also termed cryoablation, cryoneuroablation, or cryoneurolysis, is a method in which peripheral nerves are reversibly ablated by extremely cold temperatures leading to analgesia in the distribution of the nerve for multiple weeks to months. It was first reported in 1961 using liquid nitrogen to create temperatures at $-190°C$ to ablate nerves.[9,10] Lloyd and colleagues[11] coined the term "cryoanalgesia" 15 years later after describing its use for the management of pain. Since then, its clinical application expanded mainly to treat various chronic pain conditions.[12] In the few cases cryoneurolysis was used to treat acute pain, it was almost exclusively applied intraoperatively by surgically exposing the target nerves and applying the cannula under direct visualization.[13–25] More recently, cryoneurolysis was administered using a blind percutaneous approach using landmarks,[18] and subsequently using a percutaneous ultrasound-guided approach.[6,7] Most studies have involved application to sensory-only nerves. Although mixed sensory-motor nerve treatment was reported without negative sequelae in preclinical[26,27] and clinical[28] settings, its safety and therapeutic profile have yet to be determined with adequately designed and powered trials.

Mechanism of Action

The modern cryoprobe consists of a hollow tube with a smaller inner tube. Highly pressurized gas (usually nitrous oxide or carbon dioxide) travels from the proximal part of the tube to its distal portion where it is released from a larger outer tube through a narrow annulus, allowing the gas to rapidly expand in the closed tip (**Fig. 1**). Because of the Joule-Thompson effect, a drop of temperature to approximately $-70°C$ accompanies the drop in pressure, creating an ice ball at the tip of the probe.[29] The gas itself is vented back proximally through the outer tube. This mechanism ensures that no gas enters or remains in the patient's tissues.

Wallerian degeneration (a breakdown of the axon) occurs distal to the point of treatment, resulting in a complete sensory, motor, and proprioception conduction block.

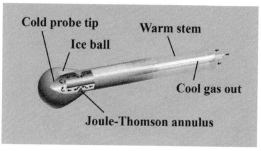

Fig. 1. A cryoneurolysis probe produces extremely cold temperature at its tip because of the Joule-Thomson effect, which results in gas flowing from a high to low pressure chamber. (*Courtesy of* B. Ilfeld, MD, MS, San Diego, CA.)

Fortunately, at temperatures warmer than −100°C, the endoneurium, perineurium, and epineurium all remain intact, permitting regeneration of the nerve of approximately 2 mm/d in a proximal-to-distal direction along the remaining nerve skeleton.[12] Cryoneurolysis using nitrous oxide or carbon dioxide has inherent safety because the freezing point of each is approximately −90°C and −80°C, and therefore each reaches a solid state before reaching −100°C, which is associated with neural and stromal destruction. Such extremely low temperatures can cause irreversible nerve injury, potentially leading to neuroma formation.[30]

Application to Acute Pain

Until recently, cryoanalgesia for acute pain management has been limited to invasive approaches that require surgical exposure of the target nerves.[24,25,31] Most of these examples target post-thoractomy pain, in which cryoanalgesia was applied to intercostal nerves by the surgeon intraoperatively.[14–17,19,20,22,23] However, technical advances now allow percutaneous administration, specifically hand-held devices with cryoprobes easily visualized with ultrasound-guidance and cleared by the FDA (**Fig. 2**).[29] Other portable devices exist that allow percutaneous administration with ultrasound guidance (**Fig. 3**). Combined with the rising expertise of ultrasound imaging among anesthesiologists and ubiquitous availability of ultrasound devices, cryoanalgesia is now a realistic intervention for acute pain management. Advantages over continuous PNB techniques include longer duration with a single application; avoidance of the risk of local anesthetic toxicity; theoretically decreased risk of infection; a lack of infusion pump malfunction, catheter migration/dislodgement, and leakage

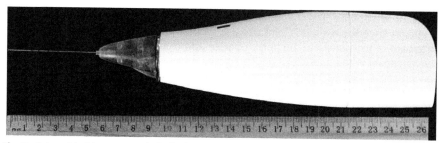

Fig. 2. A hand-held cryoneurolysis device with a 5.5-cm, 22 cryoprobe. (*Courtesy of* B. Ilfeld, MD, MS, San Diego, CA.)

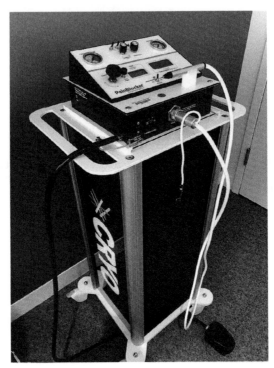

Fig. 3. A portable cryoneurolysis device with built-in nerve stimulator (PainBlocker). (*Courtesy of* B. Ilfeld, MD, MS, San Diego, CA and Epimed, Dallas, TX.)

complications; and no burden of carrying an infusion pump and local anesthetic reservoir.

Dasa and colleagues[18] were the first to analyze the efficacy of a percutaneous approach to cryoanalgesia for management of post-TKA pain. Cryoneurolysis was performed at an office visit to the surgeon days before the scheduled surgery. A blind approach used landmarks to apply percutaneous cryoanalgesia along two treatment lines to treat the anterior femoral cutaneous nerve and the infrapatellar branch of the saphenous nerve (**Fig. 4**).[32] Both nerves provide purely sensory innervation to the anterior aspect of the knee and lie in a predictable and superficial location in the proximity of the knee capsule. The anterior femoral cutaneous nerve innervating the superior knee lies within the fascia above the quadriceps tendon as it crosses a horizontal line the width of the patella approximately 7 cm above the superior aspect of the patella. The infrapatellar branch of the saphenous nerve innervating the inferior knee lies along the joint capsule and crosses a vertical line from the inferior aspect of the patella to the tibial tubercle approximately 5 cm medial to the patella. Because of the superficial and predictable locations of each of these nerves, applying cryoanalgesia using landmark techniques is possible. To block these two nerves with cryoneurolysis, Dasa and colleagues[18] applied superficial treatment with a hand-held cryodevice to produce a 0.5-cm cold zone under the skin. A treatment cycle consisted of a period of cooling then warming of the probe, lasting approximately 50 seconds. Each treatment line required approximately six treatment cycles to cover the entire length (total procedural duration to freeze both nerves was 15 minutes).

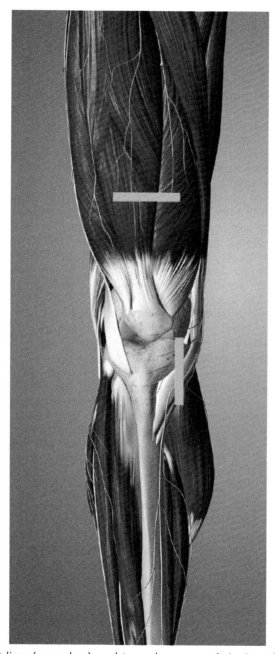

Fig. 4. Treatment lines (*green bars*) used to apply cryoneurolysis via a "blind" superficial approach to target anterior femoral cutaneous nerve and the infrapatellar branch of the saphenous nerve. (*Courtesy of* B. Ilfeld, MD, MS, San Diego, CA.)

This retrospective study of 100 patients reported the use of preoperative cryoneurolysis was associated with a reduced incidence of prolonged hospitalization duration and opioid consumption up to 12 weeks postoperatively in patients undergoing TKA.[18] Similarly, this blind approach using landmark techniques was used to treat nonsurgical pain associated with knee osteoarthritis.[33] In this randomized, double-blind, sham-controlled multicenter study, the infrapatellar branch of the saphenous nerve was targeted with cryoneurolysis. The study population consisted of 180 patients, in which those in the treatment group had statistically significant decreases from baseline Western Ontario and McMaster Osteoarthritis Index (an instrument measuring functioning) and pain scores at 30, 60, and 90 days after treatment when compared with the control group.

The use of ultrasound guidance combined with a percutaneous cryoprobe offer the ability to target far more peripheral nerves than the blind approach that is appropriate exclusively for cutaneous nerves. An ultrasound-guided percutaneous technique has been recently described but is currently limited to short series of cases.[6,7] Preoperative ultrasound-guided percutaneous cryoanalgesia for use in treating acute postoperative pain in the orthopedic population has also been reported.[7] Like the previously described reports, the infrapatellar branch was targeted by preoperative cryoneurolysis in patients planned for TKA. In contrast to prior studies, this approach used ultrasound-guidance to target the nerve versus a blind landmark technique. The case series also reports use of ultrasound guidance to visualize cryoprobe positioning and treatment of the suprascapular nerve just superior to the suprascapular notch for patients undergoing rotator cuff repair. All patients in this case series experienced excellent postoperative analgesia and had decreased opioid consumption compared with historical control subjects. No adverse events were reported.

In another report, ultrasound-guided percutaneous cryoanalgesia was used postoperatively or postinjury to treat the (1) intercostal nerve to provide multiple weeks of analgesia to a patient with refractory back pain associated with a surgical incision from a nephrolithotomy procedure; (2) subcostal and intercostal nerves to provide weeks of analgesia to a patient with hip pain following iliac crest bone grafting; and (3) the saphenous, sural, posterior tibial, and superficial peroneal nerves to help manage pain in a patient with burn injury to the foot.[6] In all cases, patients reported adequate analgesia for at least 2 weeks following treatment with no subsequent nerve injury or neuropathic pain. No other adverse events occurred in relation to cryoanalgesia.

Potential Risks

Compared with other invasive analgesic modalities, cryoanalgesia has few contraindications and risks. Relative contraindications include Reynaud syndrome, cryoglobulinemia, and cold urticaria.[34] The associated prolonged total sensory, motor, and proprioception block combined with an unpredictable duration of action (weeks to months) is not appropriate in most clinical scenarios involving acute pain with the one potential exception being the treatment of the anterior femoral cutaneous and infrapatellar branch of the saphenous nerve for knee surgery, such as knee arthroplasty.[18,32]

Similar to traditional needle-based percutaneous regional anesthesia techniques, potential complications of cryoneurolysis include bleeding, bruising, and infection. Additional risks include injury to the nerve or surrounding tissue if the cannula is retracted before resolution of the ice ball, and cutaneous discoloration if the ice ball reaches the skin.[29] Therefore, when treating superficial nerves it is important to use a cannula designed specifically for this area with heating units at and below the skin to protect against inadvertently involving the dermis and epidermis.

Of note, cryoneurolysis has been in clinical use for more than five decades without a single published case of permanent nerve injury or neuroma[28] and no evidence of long-term changes to nerve function.[26,30] However, two randomized, controlled clinical trials reported an increase in neuropathic pain associated with cryoneurolysis when administered via the surgical incision during thoracotomy.[16,19] One study compared epidural infusion alone with a combination of epidural infusion and intercostal cryoanalgesia and identified a higher incidence of neuropathic-type pain (mainly allodynia) at 8 weeks, but resolving by 6 months.[16] Furthermore, this study reports that patients who had received cryoneurolysis had higher pain scores at various time points (12 hours, 2 days, and 8 weeks). Of note, the statistical significance for this analysis was not adjusted for multiple comparisons and these results are, therefore, inconclusive. The second investigation compared epidural infusion alone with intercostal cryoanalgesia alone.[19] They reported an increased incidence of allodynia for subjects who had received cryoneurolysis at 6 and 12 months. However, statistical significance was not adjusted for multiple comparisons. Furthermore, it remains unknown if the difference in treatments was caused by an increased risk of cryoneurolysis or a protective effect from the epidural infusion.

For both studies, cryoanalgesia was applied via surgical exposure and possible nerve retraction. This is significant because preclinical evidence suggests that any physical manipulation of the nerve at the time of cryoneurolysis may be a mitigating factor in producing a sustained chronic pain condition.[35] Although not perfectly understood, the nerve manipulation before the freeze is hypothesized to produce an afferent barrage that sets up the central sensitization such that when axonal regeneration occurs following cryoneurolysis, the fiber activity is perceived as dysesthetic.[36] Although this issue certainly deserves further investigation, it is relevant that most clinical reports identified no increased risk involving thoracotomy or any other surgical procedure,[6,7,18,20,21,23–25,31,37,38] and percutaneous application does not involve nerve manipulation. Lastly, preclinical data suggest that a partial nerve injury (inducing Wallerian degeneration of only a portion of nerve fibers) results in hyperalgesia, whereas a complete ablation does not.[35] It is therefore possible that incomplete neurolysis could explain why two trials found an association between cryoanalgesia and allodynia in contrast to most similar investigations.

Summary of Cryoanalgesia

There are currently far more unresolved questions than conclusive answers regarding the use of cryoneurolysis to treat post–knee arthroplasty pain. Remaining undetermined is the optimal number of cryoneurolysis applications for each target nerve, the duration of treatment, the duration of thawing before subsequently moving the cannula, and specific apparatus and cannula design. For example, there are preclinical data suggesting that the duration of analgesia/anesthesia is directly correlated with the duration of cryoneurolysis application (30–120 seconds),[22] suggesting that the ultimate treatment duration may be better controlled than currently realized. However, additional laboratory studies have demonstrated that partial nerve injury (inducing Wallerian degeneration of only a portion of nerve fibers) results in hyperalgesia.[35] Most importantly, outcome data from randomized, controlled clinical trials are required to identify and quantify any improvement in outcomes and associated risks. This technique should be compared with local anesthetic-based analgesic modalities; however, the optimal pain control method may involve a combination of PNBs and cryoneurolysis for short- and long-term analgesia, respectively. Nonetheless, the use of cryoanalgesia for TKA patients seems promising because of the combination of few contraindications, easy technical application, new portable cryoneurolysis devices and disposable cannulas, few apparent risks, and prolonged duration that in many cases outlasts the surgical pain itself.

PERIPHERAL NEUROMODULATION

The concept of using electricity to induce analgesia is not new, having originated with the ancient Romans using living torpedo fish.[39] Since the first device designed to provide electroanalgesia became available in the early twentieth century,[40] neuromodulation has mainly evolved for the management of chronic pain through implanted spinal cord and PNS devices.[41,42] Use of PNS to treat acute postoperative pain has been limited primarily because of the invasive and time-consuming nature of the available technology.[43] Although transcutaneous delivery of electrical current has been reported, the analgesic ceiling caused by triggering pain fibers in the skin significantly limits the degree of postoperative analgesia benefit.[44] The development and FDA clearance of a lead that is inserted percutaneously through a needle has now removed the limitation of invasive surgical implantation and extraction, thus opening the possibility of applying neuromodulation to treat postoperative pain (**Fig. 5**).

Extremely small, insulated electrical leads (**Fig. 6**) have been developed that allow rapid placement via a percutaneous approach through an introducer needle.[45,46] An ultrasound-guided percutaneous approach using these extremely small leads has been used for various chronic pain states[47,48]; but, its potential for acute postoperative pain management remains primarily unexplored. Using ultrasound, these leads are placed via an introducer needle proximal to nerve (about 1–2 cm away). Unlike traditional PNB techniques, needle placement does not need to be in contact with the nerve to ensure appropriate local anesthetic spread. Stimulation is subsequently tested and if appropriate paresthesias or motor stimulation is elicited, the introducer needle is removed and lead left remaining *in situ*. The proximal portion of the lead is then attached to a small external stimulator, which can easily be affixed to the patient's skin (**Fig. 7**).[8]

Mechanism of Action

The definitive mechanism of neuromodulation's effect on pain remains unknown, although multiple theories have been proposed. The most commonly noted is "gate control theory," in which electrical activation of large-diameter myelinated afferent peripheral nerve fibers inhibits pain signals from the small-diameter pain fibers to the central nervous system.[49] The resultant effect is analgesia while preserving motor, sensory, and proprioception.

Peripheral Nerve Stimulation and Acute Pain

Ultrasound-guided percutaneous PNS offers a novel intervention to provide post–knee arthroplasty analgesia without the major limitations of opioids and continuous PNB.[8] Just one example is the associated motor, sensory, and proprioception deficits

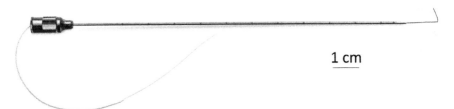

1 cm

Fig. 5. A small diameter (0.2-mm), open-coiled, helical electrical lead with an anchoring wire preloaded within a 12.5-cm, 20-gauge insertion needle for percutaneous application. (*Courtesy of* B. Ilfeld, MD, MS, San Diego, CA.)

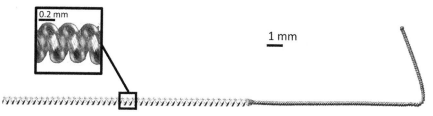

Fig. 6. A small diameter (0.2-mm), open-coiled, helical electrical lead. (*Courtesy of* B. Ilfeld, MD, MS, San Diego, CA.)

from the local anesthetic that may increase the risk of falling after joint replacement.[4] Therefore, neuromodulation has important potential implications for use in total joint surgeries because this intervention potentially may provide effective analgesia while also preserving complete motor function and proprioception, both of which are required to optimize postoperative rehabilitation and safety.

Recent preliminary studies provide data regarding the use of ultrasound-guided percutaneous lead placement and subsequent PNS in the management of acute post-operative pain following TKA.[50,51] In one pilot study, leads were placed in five subjects (femoral and/or sciatic nerve) who experienced uncontrolled postoperative pain with oral analgesics between 8 and 58 days following TKA.[50] Following lead insertion, pain scores were recorded before and after the stimulators were activated. Immediate analgesia was experienced by all subjects and decreased resting pain by an average

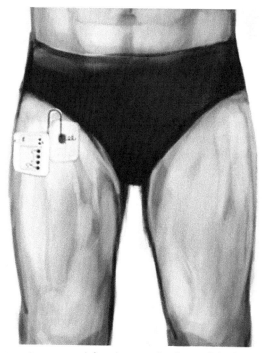

Fig. 7. Setup for a percutaneous peripheral nerve stimulator of the femoral nerve. (*Courtesy of* B. Ilfeld, MD, MS, San Diego, CA.)

of 93%, in which four of the five patients reported complete resolution of pain. Pain during passive and active knee motion was reduced by 27% and 30%, respectively, whereas maximum passive or active knee range-of-motion were only minimally affected. A second study involving another small series of subjects reported similar findings using an identical protocol between 8 and 97 days following TKA.[52]

Only a single report has been published describing the use of percutaneous PNS to treat pain in the immediate postoperative period.[53] Femoral and sciatic leads were inserted preoperatively in seven patients and remained for up to 6 weeks. During the first 2 weeks, pain was well controlled in 88% of the patients, four of whom did not require addition opioids after this time period. Of the five subjects with data on opioid use, the median time to complete opioid cessation was only 8 days, with 100% of subjects opioid-free 1 month following surgery. This is a dramatic improvement compared with the typical median time to cessation of nearly 2 months (vs 8 days)[54–57] with a 1-month opioid-independence rate of 11% to 33% (vs 100%) for patients having the same surgical procedure within the United States.[58] The average 6-minute-walk-test distance was 97% and 124% of patients' preoperative distances at 2 weeks and at 3 months, respectively. Importantly, there were no falls, motor block, or infections reported.

Potential Risks and Concerns

Potential risks associated with percutaneous PNS are, theoretically, minimal relative to current local anesthetic-based techniques; however, there have been no confirmatory large-scale clinical trials involving this novel modality. As with any implanted foreign body, there is a risk of infection. Yet the risk seems to be exceedingly low, with fewer than one infection per 3000 indwelling days,[59] orders of magnitude smaller than for perineural catheters.[60] This improvement is most likely because of the helical coil lead design, which encourages tissue ingrowth between the coils sealing the passage through the skin, and allowing stretching/compression of the lead avoiding "pistoning" that draws bacteria into the body (**Fig. 8**). Additional risks include migration, dislodgement, and fracture. As with infections, the helical coil lead design theoretically minimizes migration and dislodgement by allowing the lead to stretch and compress, unlike perineural catheters. As a result, the helical coil design permits long duration of lead retention from multiple weeks to more than a year.[61–63]

Fracture of the 2-mm diameter lead occurs in approximately 7.5% of subjects, usually during extraction, but sometimes simply during use.[8] In more than 200 patients with a fractured lead, the lead remnants were uniformly left *in situ* without any

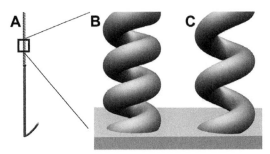

Fig. 8. Illustration showing how (*A*) electrical lead (*B*) when at rest and (*C*) when applied traction causes an opening of the helical coil, which prevents pistoning through the skin and dislodgment. (*Courtesy of* B. Ilfeld, MD, MS, San Diego, CA.)

subsequent negative sequelae.[8] Importantly, the remnants themselves do not preclude subsequent MRI.[64] Although not reported to date, there is the risk of nerve injury as with any invasive procedure. However, this risk is theoretically far lower than for local anesthetic-based PNBs considering the lead, and therefore insertion needle, do not require the lead and nerve to be in direct contact (unlike traditional PNB). Allowing for a remote distance from the nerve promotes selective stimulation of the required larger-diameter myelinated sensory neurons[65] without activating motor or smaller-diameter sensory neurons that induce muscle contraction and discomfort, respectively.[8] After 50 years of clinical use, we are unaware of any reports of nerve injury caused by the electric current of neuromodulation.[66] Many of the risks of continuous PNB do not apply to percutaneous PNS, such as local anesthetic toxicity and sensory, motor, and proprioception blockade (which may increase risk of falls). Finally, because the required external stimulator for percutaneous PNS is small and requires no medication bag to hold local anesthetic, this burden is no longer an issue with percutaneous PNS.

SUMMARY

With increased awareness of opioid overuse after surgery and the current worldwide opioid epidemic, it is timely to introduce and study novel interventions that may aid in long-term management of postsurgical pain to decrease opioid requirements. Also noteworthy is that during the first few days following knee arthroplasty, adequate analgesia improves ambulation, which is associated with shorter hospital length of stay and lower hospitalization costs.[67] Improved analgesia during the weeks to months following knee arthroplasty will theoretically aid in improved physical therapy participation and reduce opioid requirements at home.

Before ultrasound-guided percutaneous cryoanalgesia and percutaneous PNS may be more widely practiced, robust clinical trials demonstrating their efficacy in managing acute and subacute postoperative pain should be completed. Furthermore, other hospital metrics should be examined including hospital length of stay, opioid consumption, incidence of adverse events, and health care expenditures. Lastly, until the costs of percutaneous PNS systems are better defined, a cost-benefit analysis will remain inconclusive. Nevertheless, given the need to improve postoperative analgesia, decrease opioid requirements because of the current opioid epidemic, shorten hospitalization duration, improve postoperative functional outcomes, and lessen analgesic-associated patient risks, such as falling, ultrasound-guided percutaneous cryoanalgesia and PNS deserve further consideration and investigation.

ACKNOWLEDGMENTS

The authors thank Elan Ilfeld for his rendering of **Figs. 1** and **8**.

REFERENCES

1. Kopp SL, Borglum J, Buvanendran A, et al. Anesthesia and analgesia practice pathway options for total knee arthroplasty: an evidence-based review by the American and European societies of regional anesthesia and pain medicine. Reg Anesth Pain Med 2017;42(6):683–97.

2. Terkawi AS, Mavridis D, Sessler DI, et al. Pain management modalities after total knee arthroplasty: a network meta-analysis of 170 randomized controlled trials. Anesthesiology 2017;126(5):923–37.

3. Gabriel RA, Ilfeld BM. Use of regional anesthesia for outpatient surgery within the United States: a prevalence study using a nationwide database. Anesth Analg 2018;126(6):2078–84.

4. Ilfeld BM, Duke KB, Donohue MC. The association between lower extremity continuous peripheral nerve blocks and patient falls after knee and hip arthroplasty. Anesth Analg 2010;111(6):1552–4.

5. Ilfeld BM. Continuous peripheral nerve blocks: an update of the published evidence and comparison with novel, alternative analgesic modalities. Anesth Analg 2017;124(1):308–35.

6. Gabriel RA, Finneran JJ, Asokan D, et al. Ultrasound-guided percutaneous cryoneurolysis for acute pain management: a case report. A Case Rep 2017;9(5): 129–32.

7. Ilfeld BM, Gabriel RA, Trescot AM. Ultrasound-guided percutaneous cryoneurolysis providing postoperative analgesia lasting many weeks following a single administration: a replacement for continuous peripheral nerve blocks? A case report. Korean J Anesthesiol 2017;70(5):567–70.

8. Ilfeld BM, Grant SA. Ultrasound-guided percutaneous peripheral nerve stimulation for postoperative analgesia: could neurostimulation replace continuous peripheral nerve blocks? Reg Anesth Pain Med 2016;41(6):720–2.

9. Gage AA. History of cryosurgery. Semin Surg Oncol 1998;14(2):99–109.

10. Cooper IS, Grissman F, Johnston R. A complete system for cytogenic surgery. St Barnabas Hosp Med Bull 1962;1:11–6.

11. Lloyd JW, Barnard JD, Glynn CJ. Cryoanalgesia. A new approach to pain relief. Lancet 1976;2(7992):932–4.

12. Trescot AM. Cryoanalgesia in interventional pain management. Pain Physician 2003;6(3):345–60.

13. Graves C, Idowu O, Lee S, et al. Intraoperative cryoanalgesia for managing pain after the Nuss procedure. J Pediatr Surg 2017;52(6):920–4.

14. Ba YF, Li XD, Zhang X, et al. Comparison of the analgesic effects of cryoanalgesia vs. parecoxib for lung cancer patients after lobectomy. Surg Today 2015; 45(10):1250–4.

15. Sepsas E, Misthos P, Anagnostopulu M, et al. The role of intercostal cryoanalgesia in post-thoracotomy analgesia. Interact Cardiovasc Thorac Surg 2013;16(6): 814–8.

16. Mustola ST, Lempinen J, Saimanen E, et al. Efficacy of thoracic epidural analgesia with or without intercostal nerve cryoanalgesia for postthoracotomy pain. Ann Thorac Surg 2011;91(3):869–73.

17. Keller BA, Kabagambe SK, Becker JC, et al. Intercostal nerve cryoablation versus thoracic epidural catheters for postoperative analgesia following pectus excavatum repair: preliminary outcomes in twenty-six cryoablation patients. J Pediatr Surg 2016;51(12):2033–8.

18. Dasa V, Lensing G, Parsons M, et al. Percutaneous freezing of sensory nerves prior to total knee arthroplasty. Knee 2016;23(3):523–8.

19. Ju H, Feng Y, Yang BX, et al. Comparison of epidural analgesia and intercostal nerve cryoanalgesia for post-thoracotomy pain control. Eur J Pain 2008;12(3): 378–84.

20. Yang MK, Cho CH, Kim YC. The effects of cryoanalgesia combined with thoracic epidural analgesia in patients undergoing thoracotomy. Anaesthesia 2004; 59(11):1073–7.

21. Gwak MS, Yang M, Hahm TS, et al. Effect of cryoanalgesia combined with intravenous continuous analgesia in thoracotomy patients. J Korean Med Sci 2004; 19(1):74–8.

22. Moorjani N, Zhao F, Tian Y, et al. Effects of cryoanalgesia on post-thoracotomy pain and on the structure of intercostal nerves: a human prospective randomized trial and a histological study. Eur J Cardiothorac Surg 2001;20(3):502–7.

23. Bucerius J, Metz S, Walther T, et al. Pain is significantly reduced by cryoablation therapy in patients with lateral minithoracotomy. Ann Thorac Surg 2000;70(3): 1100–4.

24. Robinson SR, Purdie GL. Reducing post-tonsillectomy pain with cryoanalgesia: a randomized controlled trial. Laryngoscope 2000;110(7):1128–31.

25. Callesen T, Bech K, Thorup J, et al. Cryoanalgesia: effect on postherniorrhaphy pain. Anesth Analg 1998;87(4):896–9.

26. Hsu M, Stevenson FF. Reduction in muscular motility by selective focused cold therapy: a preclinical study. J Neural Transm (Vienna) 2014;121(1):15–20.

27. Hsu M, Stevenson FF. Wallerian degeneration and recovery of motor nerves after multiple focused cold therapies. Muscle Nerve 2015;51(2):268–75.

28. Kim PS, Ferrante FM. Cryoanalgesia: a novel treatment for hip adductor spasticity and obturator neuralgia. Anesthesiology 1998;89(2):534–6.

29. Ilfeld BM, Preciado J, Trescot AM. Novel cryoneurolysis device for the treatment of sensory and motor peripheral nerves. Expert Rev Med Devices 2016;13(8): 713–25.

30. Connelly NR, Malik A, Madabushi L, et al. Use of ultrasound-guided cryotherapy for the management of chronic pain states. J Clin Anesth 2013;25(8):634–6.

31. Wood GJ, Lloyd JW, Bullingham RE, et al. Postoperative analgesia for day-case herniorrhaphy patients. A comparison of cryoanalgesia, paravertebral blockade and oral analgesia. Anaesthesia 1981;36(6):603–10.

32. Hu E, Preciado J, Dasa V, et al. Development and validation of a new method for locating patella sensory nerves for the treatment of inferior and superior knee pain. J Exp Orthop 2015;2(1):16.

33. Radnovich R, Scott D, Patel AT, et al. Cryoneurolysis to treat the pain and symptoms of knee osteoarthritis: a multicenter, randomized, double-blind, sham-controlled trial. Osteoarthritis Cartilage 2017;25(8):1247–56.

34. Ilfeld BM, Gabriel RA, Trescot AM. Ultrasound-guided percutaneous cryoneurolysis for treatment of acute pain: could cryoanalgesia replace continuous peripheral nerve blocks? Br J Anaesth 2017;119(4):703–6.

35. Myers RR, Heckman HM, Powell HC. Axonal viability and the persistence of thermal hyperalgesia after partial freeze lesions of nerve. J Neurol Sci 1996;139(1): 28–38.

36. Wagner R, DeLeo JA, Heckman HM, et al. Peripheral nerve pathology following sciatic cryoneurolysis: relationship to neuropathic behaviors in the rat. Exp Neurol 1995;133(2):256–64.

37. Miguel R, Hubbell D. Pain management and spirometry following thoracotomy: a prospective, randomized study of four techniques. J Cardiothorac Vasc Anesth 1993;7(5):529–34.

38. Katz J, Nelson W, Forest R, et al. Cryoanalgesia for post-thoracotomy pain. Lancet 1980;1(8167):512–3.

39. Tsoucalas G, Karamanou M, Lymperi M, et al. The "torpedo" effect in medicine. Int Marit Health 2014;65(2):65–7.

40. Gildenberg PL. History of electrical neuromodulation for chronic pain. Pain Med 2006;7(1):S7–13.

41. Long DM. Electrical stimulation for relief of pain from chronic nerve injury. J Neurosurg 1973;39(6):718–22.

42. Deer TR, Mekhail N, Provenzano D, et al. The appropriate use of neurostimulation of the spinal cord and peripheral nervous system for the treatment of chronic pain and ischemic diseases: the Neuromodulation Appropriateness Consensus Committee. Neuromodulation 2014;17(6):515–50 [discussion: 550].

43. Hassenbusch SJ, Stanton-Hicks M, Schoppa D, et al. Long-term results of peripheral nerve stimulation for reflex sympathetic dystrophy. J Neurosurg 1996; 84(3):415–23.

44. Yu DT, Chae J, Walker ME, et al. Comparing stimulation-induced pain during percutaneous (intramuscular) and transcutaneous neuromuscular electric stimulation for treating shoulder subluxation in hemiplegia. Arch Phys Med Rehabil 2001;82(6):756–60.

45. Deer TR, Levy RM, Rosenfeld EL. Prospective clinical study of a new implantable peripheral nerve stimulation device to treat chronic pain. Clin J Pain 2010;26(5): 359–72.

46. Yu DT, Chae J, Walker ME, et al. Percutaneous intramuscular neuromuscular electric stimulation for the treatment of shoulder subluxation and pain in patients with chronic hemiplegia: a pilot study. Arch Phys Med Rehabil 2001;82(1):20–5.

47. Huntoon MA, Burgher AH. Ultrasound-guided permanent implantation of peripheral nerve stimulation (PNS) system for neuropathic pain of the extremities: original cases and outcomes. Pain Med 2009;10(8):1369–77.

48. Chan I, Brown AR, Park K, et al. Ultrasound-guided, percutaneous peripheral nerve stimulation: technical note. Neurosurgery 2010;67(3 Suppl Operative): ons136–9.

49. Melzack R, Wall PD. Pain mechanisms: a new theory. Science 1965;150(3699): 971–9.

50. Ilfeld BM, Gilmore CA, Grant SA, et al. Ultrasound-guided percutaneous peripheral nerve stimulation for analgesia following total knee arthroplasty: a prospective feasibility study. J Orthop Surg Res 2017;12(1):4.

51. Ilfeld BM, Ball ST, Gabriel RA, et al. Perioperative percutaneous peripheral nerve stimulation utilizing preoperative lead placement for the treatment of postoperative pain [abstract]. Reg Anesth Pain Med 2017;(3603).

52. Ilfeld BM, Grant SA, Gilmore CA, et al. Neurostimulation for postsurgical analgesia: a novel system enabling ultrasound-guided percutaneous peripheral nerve stimulation. Pain Pract 2017;17(7):892–901.

53. Ilfeld BM, Gilmore CA, Chae J, et al. Percutaneous peripheral nerve stimulation for the treatment of postoperative pain following total knee arthroplasty [abstract]. North American Neuromodulation Society conference. 2016(19:10562).

54. Namba RS, Inacio MC, Pratt NL, et al. Postoperative opioid use as an early indication of total hip arthroplasty failure. Acta Orthop 2016;87(Suppl 1):37–43.

55. Hah JM, Mackey S, Barelka PL, et al. Self-loathing aspects of depression reduce postoperative opioid cessation rate. Pain Med 2014;15(6):954–64.

56. Carroll I, Barelka P, Wang CK, et al. A pilot cohort study of the determinants of longitudinal opioid use after surgery. Anesth Analg 2012;115(3):694–702.

57. Rozet I, Nishio I, Robbertze R, et al. Prolonged opioid use after knee arthroscopy in military veterans. Anesth Analg 2014;119(2):454–9.

58. Goesling J, Moser SE, Zaidi B, et al. Trends and predictors of opioid use after total knee and total hip arthroplasty. Pain 2016;157(6):1259–65.

59. Ilfeld BM, Gabriel RA, Saulino MF, et al. Infection rates of electrical leads used for percutaneous neurostimulation of the peripheral nervous system. Pain Pract 2017;17(6):753–62.
60. Capdevila X, Bringuier S, Borgeat A. Infectious risk of continuous peripheral nerve blocks. Anesthesiology 2009;110(1):182–8.
61. Onders RP, Elmo M, Khansarinia S, et al. Complete worldwide operative experience in laparoscopic diaphragm pacing: results and differences in spinal cord injured patients and amyotrophic lateral sclerosis patients. Surg Endosc 2009; 23(7):1433–40.
62. Shimada Y, Matsunaga T, Misawa A, et al. Clinical application of peroneal nerve stimulator system using percutaneous intramuscular electrodes for correction of foot drop in hemiplegic patients. Neuromodulation 2006;9(4):320–7.
63. Marsolais EB, Kobetic R. Implantation techniques and experience with percutaneous intramuscular electrodes in the lower extremities. J Rehabil Res Dev 1986;23(3):1–8.
64. Shellock FG, Zare A, Ilfeld BM, et al. In vitro magnetic resonance imaging evaluation of fragmented, open-coil, percutaneous peripheral nerve stimulation leads. Neuromodulation 2017;21(3):276–83.
65. Grill SE, Hallett M. Velocity sensitivity of human muscle spindle afferents and slowly adapting type II cutaneous mechanoreceptors. J Physiol 1995;489(Pt 2): 593–602.
66. Mekhail NA, Cheng J, Narouze S, et al. Clinical applications of neurostimulation: forty years later. Pain Pract 2010;10(2):103–12.
67. Pua YH, Ong PH. Association of early ambulation with length of stay and costs in total knee arthroplasty: retrospective cohort study. Am J Phys Med Rehabil 2014; 93(11):962–70.

Update on Selective Regional Analgesia for Hip Surgery Patients

Dario Bugada, MD[a],*, Valentina Bellini, MD[b], Luca F. Lorini, MD[a],
Edward R. Mariano, MD, MAS (Clinical Research)[c,d]

KEYWORDS

- Total hip replacement • Hip fracture • Femoral nerve block • Fascia iliaca block
- Lumbar plexus block • Local infiltration analgesia • Surgical outcome
- Postoperative analgesia

KEY POINTS

- A wide range of selective nerve blocks are available for hip surgery analgesia, reflecting the complex innervation of the hip.
- The ideal block technique or combination for hip surgery is not yet defined; there is supportive evidence for posterior lumbar plexus, femoral nerve, and fascia iliaca blocks.
- Alternative nerve and interfascial plane blocks may have a role in analgesia for patients undergoing hip surgery but rigorous studies are lacking.
- Despite the type of block used, a strategy of multimodal analgesia in the perioperative period is mandatory.

INTRODUCTION

The hip surgery patient population worldwide is quite diverse, from children with congenital hip dysplasia, to younger athletic adults who undergo hip arthroscopy, to frail elderly patients with multiple medical problems who suffer a mechanical fall. This review focuses on adult hip surgery patients with a special emphasis on the applications of regional anesthesia and analgesia following hip fracture repair and total hip arthroplasty (THA).

[a] Emergency and Intensive Care Department, ASST Papa Giovanni XXIII, Piazza OMS, 1, Bergamo 24127, Italy; [b] Department of Anesthesia and Pain Therapy, Parma University Hospital, Via Gramsci, 14, Parma 43126, Italy; [c] Department of Anesthesiology, Perioperative and Pain Medicine, Stanford University School of Medicine, 3801 Miranda Avenue, MC 112A, Palo Alto, CA 94304, USA; [d] Anesthesiology and Perioperative Care Service, Veterans Affairs Palo Alto Health Care System, 3801 Miranda Avenue, MC 112A, Palo Alto, CA 94304, USA
* Corresponding author. Emergency and Intensive Care Department, ASST Papa Giovanni XXIII, Piazza OMS, 1, Bergamo 24127, Italy.
E-mail address: dariobugada@gmail.com

Anesthesiology Clin 36 (2018) 403–415
https://doi.org/10.1016/j.anclin.2018.04.001
1932-2275/18/© 2018 Elsevier Inc. All rights reserved.

anesthesiology.theclinics.com

Hip fracture due to mechanical falls continues to occur at a significant rate despite focused efforts on prevention.[1] Most of these patients are elderly and frail with multiple comorbidities. In this vulnerable population, early and appropriate analgesic treatment can have a strong positive influence on the trajectory of postoperative recovery.[2] Total joint replacement, including THA, is projected to become among the most common elective surgical procedures in the United States in the coming decade.[3] Effective pain management is an essential element of successful rehabilitation and enhanced recovery.[4,5] In this context, appropriate application of regional anesthesia and analgesia continues to play an important role in perioperative pain management but must be carefully balanced with the expected occurrence of lower limb motor block.[6]

Beyond the immediate postoperative period, regional anesthesia and analgesia can have potentially beneficial effects on long-term outcomes, especially on persistent postsurgical pain[7] and functional rehabilitation.[8] Continuous regional analgesia, in particular, has been extensively studied in patients who undergo total joint replacement surgery and may positively influence patient outcomes in other surgical settings.[9]

New appraisals on hip anatomy and innervation, as well as the emergence of new equipment and techniques, have increased the spectrum of possible regional anesthesia and analgesia options for anesthesiologists and pain physicians who care for hip surgery patients. This review presents the latest information on this topic, with special attention on anatomy, selective unilateral regional analgesic techniques, and outcome data.

REVIEW OF HIP INNERVATION

Hip innervation is complex with contributions from many nerve components. Birnbaum and colleagues[10] reported that the femoral nerve (FN) innervates the anterolateral capsule, and the obturator nerve (ON) innervates the anteromedial capsule. Combined innervation of the anterior capsule was often observed. The posterior and inferior parts of the hip joint capsule are innervated by the sacral plexus, consisting of branches directly from the sciatic or superior gluteal nerves, or via the sciatic nerve branch to the quadratus femoris muscle.

A histologic study of the hip joint capsule found nociceptive fibers to be predominantly present in the anterior and superolateral parts of the hip joint capsule. Neural fibers found in the posterior and inferior parts were identified as mechanoreceptors.[11] These findings support the assumption that the FNs and ONs may be the primary mediators of nociceptive pain from the hip joint, thus narrowing the focus of regional analgesic techniques.[12] However, blockade of the sacral plexus is necessary to provide surgical anesthesia, and the lateral femoral cutaneous nerve (LFCN) is also important for postoperative analgesia because it innervates the skin in the lateral part of the thigh, which is frequently involved in the surgical incision (**Fig. 1**). Although neuraxial blocks, epidurals, and spinal techniques are known to provide effective anesthesia and analgesia for hip surgery patients, they are nonselective for unilateral surgery and may be associated with undesirable side effects.[13]

SELECTIVE REGIONAL ANALGESIC TECHNIQUES FOR HIP JOINT SURGERY
Lumbar Plexus Block

Lumbar plexus block (LPB) targets the FN, LFCN, and ON as they run within the psoas major muscle. It is also known as the psoas compartment block. There are various

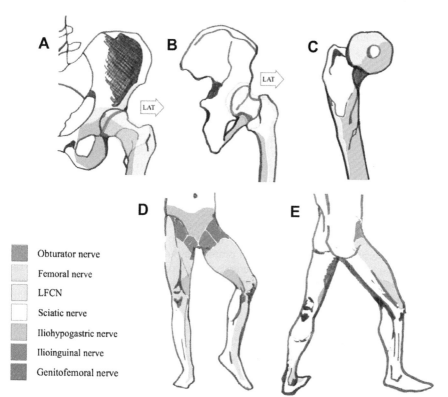

Fig. 1. Innervation of the hip joint and skin dermatomes relevant for hip surgery. Innervation: (*A*) hip joint, anterior view; (*B*) hip joint, posterior or lateral view; (*C*) femur, medial side. Skin innervation: (*D*) anterior view, (*E*) posterior view. LAT, lateral.

Legend:
- Obturator nerve
- Femoral nerve
- LFCN
- Sciatic nerve
- Iliohypogastric nerve
- Ilioinguinal nerve
- Genitofemoral nerve

approaches to perform the LPB technique using both electrical stimulation and ultrasound guidance.[14,15]

Despite the introduction of newer approaches, the use of ultrasound for LPB in adults has to date been unfortunately less helpful than in other peripheral blocks.[16] The main reason is likely the depth of the plexus, resulting in reduced image resolution and poor needle visualization. Nevertheless, the use of ultrasound imaging for pre-puncture scanning[17] or in conjunction with peripheral nerve stimulation may enhance block performance by providing an indication of psoas muscle depth, position of the kidney, and spread of injectate.[18]

The primary indication for LPB is postoperative analgesia after major hip surgery such as arthroplasty. Single-injection LPB reduces pain ratings and postoperative morphine requirements.[19] Continuous LPB results in excellent pain relief during the first 48 hours[20] and decreases the time required to achieve discharge criteria.[21] Compared with neuraxial blockade, LPB results in less hypotension and improved analgesia in elderly patients undergoing hip fracture repair[15] and is as effective as epidural block for analgesia after THA, with less nausea, urinary retention, motor block, and hypotension.

Despite proven efficacy, potential side effects and serious complications have traditionally limited the use of LPB. LPB is considered a deep block and is subject to all the restrictions of neuraxial block in the anticoagulated patient.[22,23] Further, neuraxial and bilateral spread can occur; the close proximity of the epidural and intrathecal spaces may result in catheter misplacement.[24]

These concerns are based on the findings of a major multiinstitutional study of complications after regional anesthesia that found 5 serious complications after 394 LPB procedures,[25] all either secondary to the occurrence of intrathecal or epidural block, or intravascular local anesthetic administration. A more recent registry confirms that severe complications are still possible despite all precautions related to the prevention of neuraxial spread and intravascular injection.[26] The reason for the migration of injectate is not completely understood but it is thought that it relies on the diffusion along nerve roots toward the neuraxis. Various attempts have been made to reduce this phenomenon but neuraxial spread of local anesthetic can still occur in up to 30% of cases. The technique used for LPB,[27] use of ultrasound, and the reduction in the volume of local anesthetics do not seem to eliminate the problem.[28] Recently, severe complications have been associated with even the lowest possible volumes of injectate to obtain a successful LPB; therefore, 100% prevention may not be possible even with new ultrasound-guided approaches.[26,28] Only limiting opening injection pressure (<15 psi)[24] and lateral position[29] seem to be protective but no large prospective studies are available to support this claim. Hemodynamic monitoring, therefore, should be continued for 45 minutes after block with regular assessment for contralateral spread by sensory testing. Use of a test dose and/or radiological imaging may be warranted to confirm catheter placement.[30]

In a randomized clinical trial (RCT) comparing continuous LPB to a proximally inserted FN catheter technique (nearly identical to the fascia iliaca catheter) for subjects undergoing THA, postoperative analgesia was equivalent between the 2 groups.[31] Given these results and the comparison of procedure-related risks, the indications for LPB seem to be shrinking.

Fascia Iliaca Block

The concept of fascia iliaca block (FIB) is to introduce high volumes of local anesthetic underneath the fascia iliaca, assuming that the proximal diffusion of the injectate along the psoas muscle will target FNs, LFCNs, and ONs during their course (the so-called 3-in-1 block).

Different techniques are available. The first to be described was the landmark-based double-pop technique,[32] a loss-of-resistance approach based on the pop felt when the needle passes through both fascia lata and fascia iliaca.

Ultrasound-guided approaches have also been described. One early approach recommends the use of high frequency linear transducer with transverse orientation placed below the inguinal ligament and lateral to the femoral artery. A more cranial access point (above the inguinal ligament) has been described[33] in the attempt to increase proximal local anesthetic spread to the iliac fossa. The orientation of the probe seems to influence block success with perpendicular orientation to the inguinal ligament associated with greater incidence of successful LFCN block.[34] Without ultrasound, the accuracy of the loss-of-resistance technique in positioning the needle in the fascia iliaca compartment is 56%, with drug diffusion above the fascia in 14% and intramuscular injection in 29% of patients.[35] Ultrasound guidance increases the frequency of FN block (FNB) and ON block (ONB).[36]

When compared with the FNB technique, FIB may have an inherent safety advantage because the puncture site is further away from large vessels and the FN. FIB is a valuable technique that can be used in the emergency department (ED) to treat pain associated with hip fractures. RCTs have shown a statistically significant improvement in maximum pain relief both at rest and at movement,[37] with fewer adverse events compared with other analgesics.[38] Furthermore, in a recent study on ED patients with hip fracture, FIB provided immediate pain relief and allowed a larger proportion of patients to reach a clinically meaningful decrease in pain without opioids at 4 to 8 hours.[39] FIB's opioid-sparing effect and analgesic efficacy with fewer side effects have been consistently reported.[40,41]

Single-injection FIB techniques may provide effective analgesia for several hours or even up to 2 days.[42] When indicated (eg, when longer time is expected to pass between hospital admission and surgery), a catheter can be inserted to perform continuous regional analgesia with potential benefits on patient outcomes, especially cognitive impairment.[43]

FIB is also a valuable element of multimodal analgesia after THA. Despite some conflicting results, FIB has generally been shown to be superior to placebo for postoperative analgesia, irrespective of the type of hip surgery.[44,45] In a recent RCT, a high-dose longitudinal suprainguinal ultrasound-guided FIB resulted in a statistically significant reduction in morphine consumption at 24 and 48 hours postoperatively compared with intravenous analgesia alone, with decreased pain scores up to 24 hours postoperatively.[46] Continuous FIB maintained for the first 48 hours after surgery reduces pain intensity when compared with fentanyl intravenous patient-controlled analgesia, with a lower incidence of postoperative nausea and vomiting, and pruritus.[47] When managed appropriately (ie, pausing infusions hours before anticipated mobility), continuous FIB may not impair ambulatory ability for postoperative THA patients.[48]

A recent meta-analysis comparing FNB and FIB indicates that both techniques minimize opioid consumption in patients after THA.[49] A study by Rashiq and colleagues[50] compared multiple pain treatment options for subjects following hip fracture surgery, with variable timing of block execution and type of injection (eg, single-injection, catheter with continuous infusion, intermittent bolus). FIB was the most protective against postoperative delirium. Further studies are required to confirm these results.

Femoral Nerve Block

FNB is a common peripheral nerve block procedure, carries a low risk of complications, and has multiple clinical applications for postoperative analgesia. All available techniques are based on the relationship of FN to the vessels in the femoral triangle. The FN is always lateral to the artery; identifying the femoral artery (either by palpation or by ultrasound) is a helpful guide when locating the nerve. The nerve is easily identified by ultrasound (in between the fascia iliaca and iliacus muscle) and usually appears as a flat or teardrop-shaped hyperechoic structure. If using nerve stimulation, needle-to-nerve proximity is indicated by eliciting quadriceps contraction with patellar movement (the so-called dancing patella). Different approaches have been used for ultrasound-guided FNB, typically with short-axis target imaging and either out-of-plane or in-plane needle guidance.[51]

For patients presenting to the ED with acute hip pain from a proximal femoral fracture, both nerve stimulator and ultrasound guidance result in successful blocks of similar duration; however, ultrasound decreases block performance time.[52] Providing early FNB in this setting effectively controls pain during radiological examinations and traction application.[53] A recent review emphasizes FNB's effectiveness versus opioids and its higher safety profile in patients with hip fractures.[54]

FNB may also be useful when positioning patients for neuraxial anesthesia; when compared with intravenous fentanyl, FNB reduces the need for additional analgesics and decreases the time needed to perform spinal anesthesia.[55]

Single-injection FNB, although limited in duration, may offer some benefits during postoperative recovery after hip surgery. When compared with placebo, FNB can extend the time from anesthetic emergence to the first request for analgesia.[56] According to a study by Wiesmann and colleagues,[57] subjects who received an FNB for hip surgery demonstrated decreased systemic analgesic consumption up to 24 hours after surgery, improved pulmonary function, and faster achievement of postanesthesia care unit discharge criteria.

Continuous FNB provides extended postoperative analgesia after hip surgery. When a catheter is properly placed next to the FN, effective analgesic duration is longer, and the quality of analgesia is equivalent to that of a continuous LPB. A successful FNB results in quadriceps weakness,[58] which may impair early ambulatory ability after lower extremity surgery.[31] However, peripheral nerve blocks may not be entirely to blame in terms of increased fall risk. Large-scale database studies and RCTs have shown other factors (ie, obesity, age, higher comorbidity burden) to be associated with postoperative falls and difficulty with ambulation after hip arthroplasty.[48,59] For outpatient hip surgery (eg, arthroscopy), routine FNB may not be recommended due to this risk.[60] Careful consideration of risks and benefits should always be performed when evaluating potential candidates for peripheral nerve blockade, and explicit instructions regarding safe care of the affected extremity should be provided to the patient and caregivers.[61]

OTHER PERIPHERAL NERVE BLOCK TECHNIQUES
Obturator Nerve Block

The ON descends through psoas major and extends to the anterior thigh through the obturator canal. The common ON runs between the pectineus and obturator externus muscles immediately after the nerve emerges from the obturator canal. The articular branch supplying the hip joint is derived from the common ON or its branches at different levels in conjunction with the obturator canal.[62]

ONB can be performed by different techniques. Regardless of technique used, the aim for successful analgesia of the hip joint should be the common ON before bifurcation into anterior and posterior branches. When using nerve stimulation alone, blind needle advancement toward intrapelvic components may result in a higher rate of complications[63] and articular branches to the hip joint are not always blocked. Ultrasound-guided ONB below the inguinal ligament is an easy technique to block anterior and posterior divisions[64] but articular branches to the hip may be inconsistently anesthetized. Recently, a cadaveric study has demonstrated that injection of 15 mL within the muscular plane between the pectineus and the external obturator muscle provides 100% block of the articular branches.[12]

It remains unclear whether an ONB alone can significantly improve the management of acute pain after hip surgery. An RCT demonstrating equivalent analgesia between continuous FNB (essentially a fascia iliaca catheter technique) and continuous LPB[31] argues against a clinically meaningful benefit of ONB. One RCT described the combination of ONB and LFCN blockade as an effective approach in controlling acute pain after surgery for hip fracture.[52] However, the available evidence is based on indirect multicomparison analysis and should be carefully interpreted. The clinical relevance of adding ONB to a standard FNB for analgesia in hip fracture or hip surgery, or possible advantages of selective ONB compared with other plexus or peripheral nerve blocks are unclear. As understanding of hip innervation increases and the expectations for postoperative ambulation after joint replacement change, combined with advances in ultrasound-guided techniques,[65] there may yet be an indication for ONB in this setting.

Lateral Femoral Cutaneous Nerve Block

The LFCN is a sensory branch of the lumbar plexus. The LFCN divides into several branches and provides superficial innervation over the anterolateral thigh. There is a large variation in the area of sensory coverage among individuals because of the highly variable course of the LFCN and its branches. Different anatomic variants have been shown,[66] which must be taken into account when this nerve block is performed, making it challenging to perform an effective landmark-based block. Ultrasound guidance, however, allows for more accurate needle insertion into the appropriate fascial plane. The LFCN is typically visualized with ultrasound between the tensor fasciae latae and the sartorius muscles, 1 to 2 cm medial and inferior to the anterior superior iliac spine, as an oval hypoechoic small structure with a hyperechoic rim.[67]

LFCN block can be helpful for postoperative pain management in hip surgery patients but with limited effectiveness when performed alone. Thybo and colleagues[68] demonstrated that ultrasound-guided LFCN block performed postoperatively in THA subjects experiencing pain scores higher than 40 mm during hip flexion, may reduce pain at mobilization by an average of 17 mm. However, they showed a significant percentage of nonresponders (around 42%). The same investigators performed an additional RCT in which an ultrasound-guided LFCN block was administered at the end of THA, before the spinal block resolved. No differences were reported in the following 24 hours in terms of opioid consumption, pain at rest and movement, time to first mobilization, and degree of mobilization.[69] The limited effectiveness of LFCN block when performed alone may be due to the surgical incision (at least in part) extending beyond the skin area innervated by LFCN. In a group of 20 volunteers, more than half of incisions drawn according to a simulated hip arthroplasty fell completely outside the area of anesthesia produced by LFCN block. In these cases, an alternative approach may be the infiltration of the skin performed by the surgeon because LFCN selectively innervates the skin surface.[70]

Interfascial Plane Blocks: Quadratus Lumborum Block

The quadratus lumborum block (QLB) aims to block the anterior branches of thoracoabdominal nerves and may extend to the upper branches of the lumbar plexus and lateral cutaneous branches of the thoracoabdominal nerves with possible spread of injectate to the paravertebral space. Multiple approaches are described in the literature: lateral, posterior, and anterior (transmuscular). Different approaches determine different spread patterns of injectate with affected dermatomes ranging from thoracic (T)6 to lumbar (L)2.[71]

QLB has mostly been described for abdominal surgery[71] but has also recently been applied for hip fracture patients. In patients with neck of femur fracture, QLB may result in better pain control in the first 24 hours after surgery compared with FNB with a lower use of opioids.[72] La Colla and colleagues[73] have described QLB with block duration of about 30 hours, extending through T10 to L3 dermatomes, and without associated muscle weakness. Analgesia lasting more than 24 hours has been reported without association with hip flexor or quadriceps weakness in 2 other patients receiving hip surgery with 0.5% ropivacaine.[74] A continuous QLB with catheter placement may represent an option for continuous regional analgesia. In a report, 0.2% ropivacaine was infused at 7 mL per hour to provide analgesia without motor block in a single case of primary THA through posterior approach.[75]

However, not all QLB approaches are the same and motor weakness is possible,[76] especially with deeper injection of local anesthetic anterior to the quadratus lumborum muscle. With deeper approaches, considerations related to regional anesthesia in the anticoagulated patient are relevant.

There may be a role for QLB in multimodal pain management for hip surgery patients due to its potential for analgesic effectiveness and preservation of muscle strength with certain techniques, which makes it less likely to impair early functional rehabilitation. More outcome data based on prospective studies are still needed, as well as better understanding of the applications of the various QLB techniques. Safety issues should be addressed because they may limit QLB application, especially in the anticoagulated patient.

LOCAL INFILTRATION ANALGESIA

Local infiltration analgesia (LIA) relies on the injection of local anesthetic (alone or in combination with other analgesics) within the surgical field in multiple layers, providing analgesia without any motor block. In contrast to LIA for total knee replacement, which is strongly supported, the efficacy of LIA for analgesia after THA is not as widely accepted.[77,78] However, a recent RCT provides supportive evidence for the analgesic effectiveness of LIA with liposomal bupivacaine after THA.[79] Compared with intrathecal morphine and epidural analgesia, LIA was reported to have similar or improved analgesic efficacy.[80] In a recent meta-analysis, no difference was observed between LIA and peripheral nerve blocks (LPB, FNB, FIB) in terms of cumulative opioid use and pain scores at 24 hours after surgery. LIA had a greater probability of being ranked first in efficacy for patient outcomes.[81] This was confirmed by a recent study that showed higher incidence of motor block for FNB, whereas lower morphine consumption and better pain control at 24 hours were obtained with LIA; however, issues with study design may limit generalizability of these results.[82] In another recent RCT, the investigators found a modest improvement with respect to analgesia in patients receiving continuous LPB compared with those receiving LIA with ropivacaine.[79] LIA for THA requires systematic, extensive, and meticulous multilayer tissue injection before surgical wound closure, encompassing both capsular and soft tissues.[83] Injectate typically contains local anesthetics, as well as other analgesic adjuncts.[84]

SUMMARY

Hip surgery is widely performed and regional anesthesia techniques offer many benefits in terms of postoperative pain management and functional recovery. To date, no single technique or combination of techniques has been shown to be superior in all hip surgeries. Use of LPB, FNB, and FIB within the context of a multimodal regimen are all fairly well supported by published evidence. Other techniques, such as ONB and LFCN block, have limited applications when used alone. Newer regional analgesic approaches, such as QLB, still require rigorous comparative effectiveness studies against established techniques. Regardless of which block technique is used, a multimodal approach must be used. To realize potential long-term outcome benefits, more work is needed to advance postoperative regional analgesia tailored to the individual patient, beyond the first 1 to 3 days after hip surgery.

REFERENCES

1. Bhimjiyani A, Neuburger J, Jones T, et al. The effect of social deprivation on hip fracture incidence in England has not changed over 14 years: an analysis of the English Hospital Episodes Statistics (2001-2015). Osteoporos Int 2018;29(1): 115–24.

2. Centre NCG. The management of hip fracture in adults. London: National Clinical Guideline Centre; 2011.

3. Maradit Kremers H, Larson DR, Crowson CS, et al. Prevalence of total hip and knee replacement in the United States. J Bone Joint Surg Am 2015;97(17): 1386–97.

4. Andersen LO, Gaarn-Larsen L, Kristensen BB, et al. Subacute pain and function after fast-track hip and knee arthroplasty. Anaesthesia 2009;64(5):508–13.

5. Kehlet H, Soballe K. Fast-track hip and knee replacement–what are the issues? Acta Orthop 2010;81(3):271–2.

6. Shin JJ, McCrum CL, Mauro CS, et al. Pain management after hip arthroscopy: systematic review of randomized controlled trials and cohort studies. Am J Sports Med 2017. [Epub ahead of print].

7. Bugada D, Lavand'homme P, Ambrosoli AL, et al. Effect of preoperative inflammatory status and comorbidities on pain resolution and persistent postsurgical pain after inguinal hernia repair. Mediators Inflamm 2016;2016:5830347.

8. Bugada D, Allegri M, Gemma M, et al. The effects of anaesthesia and analgesia on long-term outcome after total knee replacement: a prospective, observational, multicentre study. Eur J Anaesthesiol 2017;34(10):665–72.

9. Bugada D, Ghisi D, Mariano ER. Continuous regional anesthesia: a review of perioperative outcome benefits. Minerva Anestesiol 2017;83(10):1089–100.

10. Birnbaum K, Prescher A, Hessler S, et al. The sensory innervation of the hip joint–an anatomical study. Surg Radiol Anat 1997;19(6):371–5.

11. Gerhardt M, Johnson K, Atkinson R, et al. Characterisation and classification of the neural anatomy in the human hip joint. Hip Int 2012;22(1):75–81.

12. Nielsen TD, Moriggl B, Soballe K, et al. A cadaveric study of ultrasound-guided subpectineal injectate spread around the obturator nerve and its hip articular branches. Reg Anesth Pain Med 2017;42(3):357–61.

13. Rawal N. Current issues in postoperative pain management. Eur J Anaesthesiol 2016;33(3):160–71.

14. Awad IT, Duggan EM. Posterior lumbar plexus block: anatomy, approaches, and techniques. Reg Anesth Pain Med 2005;30(2):143–9.

15. Nielsen MV, Bendtsen TF, Borglum J. Superiority of ultrasound guided Shamrock lumbar plexus block. Minerva Anestesiol 2018;84(1):115–21.

16. Kirchmair L, Entner T, Kapral S, et al. Ultrasound guidance for the psoas compartment block: an imaging study. Anesth Analg 2002;94(3):706–10 [Table of contents].

17. Ilfeld BM, Loland VJ, Mariano ER. Prepuncture ultrasound imaging to predict transverse process and lumbar plexus depth for psoas compartment block and perineural catheter insertion: a prospective, observational study. Anesth Analg 2010;110(6):1725–8.

18. Karmakar MK, Li JW, Kwok WH, et al. Ultrasound-guided lumbar plexus block using a transverse scan through the lumbar intertransverse space: a prospective case series. Reg Anesth Pain Med 2015;40(1):75–81.

19. Stevens RD, Van Gessel E, Flory N, et al. Lumbar plexus block reduces pain and blood loss associated with total hip arthroplasty. Anesthesiology 2000;93(1): 115–21.

20. Capdevila X, Macaire P, Dadure C, et al. Continuous psoas compartment block for postoperative analgesia after total hip arthroplasty: new landmarks, technical guidelines, and clinical evaluation. Anesth Analg 2002;94(6):1606–13 [Table of contents].

21. Ilfeld BM, Le LT, Meyer RS, et al. Ambulatory continuous femoral nerve blocks decrease time to discharge readiness after tricompartment total knee arthroplasty: a randomized, triple-masked, placebo-controlled study. Anesthesiology 2008;108(4):703–13.

22. Horlocker TT, Wedel DJ, Rowlingson JC, et al. Regional anesthesia in the patient receiving antithrombotic or thrombolytic therapy: American Society of Regional Anesthesia and Pain Medicine Evidence-Based Guidelines (Third Edition). Reg Anesth Pain Med 2010;35(1):64–101.

23. Dario Bugada MA, Zadra N, Antonio Braschi A, et al, RICALOR Group Investigators. Regional anesthesia and anticoagulant drugs: a survey of current Italian practice. Eur J Pain Suppl 2011;5:335–43.

24. Gadsden JC, Lindenmuth DM, Hadzic A, et al. Lumbar plexus block using high-pressure injection leads to contralateral and epidural spread. Anesthesiology 2008;109(4):683–8.

25. Auroy Y, Benhamou D, Bargues L, et al. Major complications of regional anesthesia in France: the SOS regional anesthesia hotline service. Anesthesiology 2002;97(5):1274–80.

26. Allegri M, Bugada D, Grossi P, et al. Italian Registry of Complications associated with Regional Anesthesia (RICALOR). An incidence analysis from a prospective clinical survey. Minerva Anestesiol 2016;82(4):392–402.

27. Mannion S, O'Callaghan S, Walsh M, et al. In with the new, out with the old? Comparison of two approaches for psoas compartment block. Anesth Analg 2005; 101(1):259–64 [Table of contents].

28. Sauter AR, Ullensvang K, Niemi G, et al. The Shamrock lumbar plexus block: a dose-finding study. Eur J Anaesthesiol 2015;32(11):764–70.

29. Jankowski CJ, Hebl JR, Stuart MJ, et al. A comparison of psoas compartment block and spinal and general anesthesia for outpatient knee arthroscopy. Anesth Analg 2003;97(4):1003–9 [Table of contents].

30. Mannion S. Psoas compartment block. Continuing Education Anaesth Crit Care Pain 2007;7:162–6.

31. Ilfeld BM, Mariano ER, Madison SJ, et al. Continuous femoral versus posterior lumbar plexus nerve blocks for analgesia after hip arthroplasty: a randomized, controlled study. Anesth Analg 2011;113(4):897–903.

32. Diwan S. Fascia iliaca block- an anatomical and technical description. Journal of Anaesthesia and Critical Care Case Reports 2015;1(1):27–30.

33. Hebbard P, Ivanusic J, Sha S. Ultrasound-guided supra-inguinal fascia iliaca block: a cadaveric evaluation of a novel approach. Anaesthesia 2011;66(4): 300–5.

34. Wang N, Li M, Wei Y, et al. A comparison of two approaches to ultrasound-guided fascia iliaca compartment block for analgesia after total hip arthroplasty. Zhonghua Yi Xue Za Zhi 2015;95(28):2277–81 [in Chinese].

35. Liang-Jing Yuan JY, Xu Li, Qing-Guo Y. Clinical research on loss of resistance technique in fascia iliaca compartment block. Biomed Res 2016;27(4):1082–6.

36. Dolan J, Williams A, Murney E, et al. Ultrasound guided fascia iliaca block: a comparison with the loss of resistance technique. Reg Anesth Pain Med 2008; 33(6):526–31.

37. Foss NB, Kristensen BB, Bundgaard M, et al. Fascia iliaca compartment blockade for acute pain control in hip fracture patients: a randomized, placebo-controlled trial. Anesthesiology 2007;106(4):773–8.

38. Godoy Monzon D, Vazquez J, Jauregui JR, et al. Pain treatment in post-traumatic hip fracture in the elderly: regional block vs. systemic non-steroidal analgesics. Int J Emerg Med 2010;3(4):321–5.
39. Groot L, Dijksman LM, Simons MP, et al. Single fascia iliaca compartment block is safe and effective for emergency pain relief in hip-fracture patients. West J Emerg Med 2015;16(7):1188–93.
40. Shelley BG, Haldane GJ. Pneumoretroperitoneum as a consequence of fascia iliaca block. Reg Anesth Pain Med 2006;31(6):582–3.
41. Kassam AM, Gough AT, Davies J, et al. Can we reduce morphine use in elderly, proximal femoral fracture patients using a fascia iliac block? Geriatr Nurs 2018; 39(1):84–7.
42. Levente BZ, Filip MN, Romaniuc N, et al. Efficacy and duration of ultrasound guided fascia iliaca block for hip fracture performed in the emergency departments. Rom J Anaesth Intensive Care 2017;24(2):167–9.
43. Odor PM, Chis Ster I, Wilkinson I, et al. Effect of admission fascia iliaca compartment blocks on post-operative abbreviated mental test scores in elderly fractured neck of femur patients: a retrospective cohort study. BMC Anesthesiol 2017; 17(1):2.
44. Goitia Arrola L, Telletxea S, Martinez Bourio R, et al. Fascia iliaca compartment block for analgesia following total hip replacement surgery. Rev Esp Anestesiol Reanim 2009;56(6):343–8 [in Spanish].
45. Kumie FT, Gebremedhn EG, Tawuye HY. Efficacy of fascia iliaca compartment nerve block as part of multimodal analgesia after surgery for femoral bone fracture. World J Emerg Med 2015;6(2):142–6.
46. Desmet M, Vermeylen K, Van Herreweghe I, et al. A longitudinal supra-inguinal fascia iliaca compartment block reduces morphine consumption after total hip arthroplasty. Reg Anesth Pain Med 2017;42(3):327–33.
47. Nie H, Yang YX, Wang Y, et al. Effects of continuous fascia iliaca compartment blocks for postoperative analgesia in patients with hip fracture. Pain Res Manag 2015;20(4):210–2.
48. Mudumbai SC, Kim TE, Howard SK, et al. An ultrasound-guided fascia iliaca catheter technique does not impair ambulatory ability within a clinical pathway for total hip arthroplasty. Korean J Anesthesiol 2016;69(4):368–75.
49. Fei D, Ma LP, Yuan HP, et al. Comparison of femoral nerve block and fascia iliaca block for pain management in total hip arthroplasty: a meta-analysis. Int J Surg 2017;46:11–3.
50. Rashiq S, Vandermeer B, Abou-Setta AM, et al. Efficacy of supplemental peripheral nerve blockade for hip fracture surgery: multiple treatment comparison. Can J Anaesth 2013;60(3):230–43.
51. Ruiz A, Sala-Blanch X, Martinez-Ocon J, et al. Incidence of intraneural needle insertion in ultrasound-guided femoral nerve block: a comparison between the out-of-plane versus the in-plane approaches. Rev Esp Anestesiol Reanim 2014; 61(2):73–7.
52. Forouzan A, Masoumi K, Motamed H, et al. Nerve stimulator versus ultrasound-guided femoral nerve block; a randomized clinical trial. Emerg (Tehran) 2017; 5(1):e54.
53. Somvanshi M, Tripathi A, Meena N. Femoral nerve block for acute pain relief in fracture shaft femur in an emergency ward. Saudi J Anaesth 2015;9(4):439–41.
54. Riddell M, Ospina M, Holroyd-Leduc JM. Use of femoral nerve blocks to manage hip fracture pain among older adults in the emergency department: a systematic review. CJEM 2016;18(4):245–52.

55. Hartmann FV, Novaes MR, de Carvalho MR. Femoral nerve block versus intravenous fentanyl in adult patients with hip fractures - a systematic review. Braz J Anesthesiol 2017;67(1):67–71.

56. Fournier R, Van Gessel E, Gaggero G, et al. Postoperative analgesia with "3-in-1" femoral nerve block after prosthetic hip surgery. Can J Anaesth 1998;45(1):34–8.

57. Wiesmann T, Steinfeldt T, Wagner G, et al. Supplemental single shot femoral nerve block for total hip arthroplasty: impact on early postoperative care, pain management and lung function. Minerva Anestesiol 2014;80(1):48–57.

58. Charous MT, Madison SJ, Suresh PJ, et al. Continuous femoral nerve blocks: varying local anesthetic delivery method (bolus versus basal) to minimize quadriceps motor block while maintaining sensory block. Anesthesiology 2011;115(4): 774–81.

59. Memtsoudis SG, Danninger T, Rasul R, et al. Inpatient falls after total knee arthroplasty: the role of anesthesia type and peripheral nerve blocks. Anesthesiology 2014;120(3):551–63.

60. Xing JG, Abdallah FW, Brull R, et al. Preoperative femoral nerve block for hip arthroscopy: a randomized, triple-masked controlled trial. Am J Sports Med 2015;43(11):2680–7.

61. Memtsoudis SG, Poeran J, Cozowicz C, et al. The impact of peripheral nerve blocks on perioperative outcome in hip and knee arthroplasty-a population-based study. Pain 2016;157(10):2341–9.

62. Anagnostopoulou S, Kostopanagiotou G, Paraskeuopoulos T, et al. Anatomic variations of the obturator nerve in the inguinal region: implications in conventional and ultrasound regional anesthesia techniques. Reg Anesth Pain Med 2009; 34(1):33–9.

63. Obturator nerve block. Available at: https://www.nysora.com/obturator-nerve-block. Accessed February 6, 2018.

64. Manassero A, Bossolasco M, Ugues S, et al. Ultrasound-guided obturator nerve block: interfascial injection versus a neurostimulation-assisted technique. Reg Anesth Pain Med 2012;37(1):67–71.

65. Yoshida T, Nakamoto T, Kamibayashi T. Ultrasound-guided obturator nerve block: a focused review on anatomy and updated techniques. Biomed Res Int 2017; 2017:7023750.

66. Tomaszewski KA, Popieluszko P, Henry BM, et al. The surgical anatomy of the lateral femoral cutaneous nerve in the inguinal region: a meta-analysis. Hernia 2016;20(5):649–57.

67. Hadzic A. Hadzic's peripheral nerve blocks and anatomy for ultrasound-guided regional anesthesia. 2nd edition. New York: McGraw-Hill; 2011.

68. Thybo KH, Mathiesen O, Dahl JB, et al. Lateral femoral cutaneous nerve block after total hip arthroplasty: a randomised trial. Acta Anaesthesiol Scand 2016; 60(9):1297–305.

69. Thybo KH, Schmidt H, Hagi-Pedersen D. Effect of lateral femoral cutaneous nerve-block on pain after total hip arthroplasty: a randomised, blinded, placebo-controlled trial. BMC Anesthesiol 2016;16:21.

70. Davies A, Crossley A, Harper M, et al. Lateral cutaneous femoral nerve blockade-limited skin incision coverage in hip arthroplasty. Anaesth Intensive Care 2014; 42(5):625–30.

71. Ueshima H, Otake H, Lin JA. Ultrasound-guided quadratus lumborum block: an updated review of anatomy and techniques. Biomed Res Int 2017;2017:2752876.

72. Parras T, Blanco R. Randomised trial comparing the transversus abdominis plane block posterior approach or quadratus lumborum block type I with femoral block

for postoperative analgesia in femoral neck fracture, both ultrasound-guided. Rev Esp Anestesiol Reanim 2016;63(3):141–8.

73. La Colla L, Uskova A, Ben-David B. Single-shot quadratus lumborum block for postoperative analgesia after minimally invasive hip arthroplasty: a new alternative to continuous lumbar plexus block? Reg Anesth Pain Med 2017;42(1):125–6.

74. La Colla L, Ben-David B, Merman R. Quadratus lumborum block as an alternative to lumbar plexus block for hip surgery: a report of 2 cases. A A Case Rep 2017; 8(1):4–6.

75. Hockett MM, Hembrador S, Lee A. Continuous quadratus lumborum block for postoperative pain in total hip arthroplasty: a case report. A A Case Rep 2016; 7(6):129–31.

76. Wikner M. Unexpected motor weakness following quadratus lomborum block for gynaecological laparoscopy. Anesthesia 2017;72(2):230–2.

77. Lunn TH, Husted H, Solgaard S, et al. Intraoperative local infiltration analgesia for early analgesia after total hip arthroplasty: a randomized, double-blind, placebo-controlled trial. Reg Anesth Pain Med 2011;36(5):424–9.

78. Andersen LO, Kehlet H. Analgesic efficacy of local infiltration analgesia in hip and knee arthroplasty: a systematic review. Br J Anaesth 2014;113(3):360–74.

79. Johnson RL, Amundson AW, Abdel MP, et al. Continuous posterior lumbar plexus nerve block versus periarticular injection with ropivacaine or liposomal bupivacaine for total hip arthroplasty: a three-arm randomized clinical trial. J Bone Joint Surg Am 2017;99(21):1836–45.

80. Kuchalik J, Granath B, Ljunggren A, et al. Postoperative pain relief after total hip arthroplasty: a randomized, double-blind comparison between intrathecal morphine and local infiltration analgesia. Br J Anaesth 2013;111(5):793–9.

81. Jimenez-Almonte JH, Wyles CC, Wyles SP, et al. Is local infiltration analgesia superior to peripheral nerve blockade for pain management after THA: a network meta-analysis. Clin Orthop Relat Res 2016;474(2):495–516.

82. Kuchalik J, Magnuson A, Lundin A, et al. Local infiltration analgesia or femoral nerve block for postoperative pain management in patients undergoing total hip arthroplasty. A randomized, double-blind study. Scand J Pain 2017;16: 223–30.

83. Joshi GP, Cushner FD, Barrington JW, et al. Techniques for periarticular infiltration with liposomal bupivacaine for the management of pain after hip and knee arthroplasty: a consensus recommendation. J Surg Orthop Adv 2015;24(1):27–35.

84. Ross JA, Greenwood AC, Sasser P 3rd, et al. Periarticular injections in knee and hip arthroplasty: where and what to inject. J Arthroplasty 2017;32(9s):S77–80.

Enhanced Recovery After Shoulder Arthroplasty

Taras Grosh, MD*, Nabil M. Elkassabany, MD, MSCE

KEYWORDS

- Shoulder arthroplasty • Enhanced recovery after surgery • Multimodal analgesia
- Regional anesthesia • Perineural catheter • Perioperative surgical home

KEY POINTS

- Enhanced recovery protocols in joint arthroplasty reduce morbidity and mortality, readmission rates, and length of stay while improving analgesia and patient satisfaction.
- Protocols for shoulder arthroplasty demonstrate benefits similar to lower extremity arthroplasty based on preliminary data.
- Despite success, universal protocol adoption is lacking.
- Future protocols must focus on patient-centered metrics and functional outcomes beyond the immediate postoperative period.

INTRODUCTION

Enhanced recovery after surgery (ERAS) is a patient-centered, evidence-based, multidisciplinary collaborative management approach that charts a patient's course before, during, and after surgery.[1] ERAS should be procedure-specific; based on the recovery goals after each type of surgery; and designed with aims to decrease the perioperative stress response, optimize patients' physiologic function, and speed recovery.[2] The first ERAS protocols started in colorectal surgery, but ERAS now includes almost all surgical subspecialties, including orthopedic surgery. Joint arthroplasty surgeries are costly not only to the patient but also to the health care system.[3] Although total joint arthroplasty equipment, techniques, and the concomitant anesthesia have evolved, complications leading to significant physiologic derangements still occur. This departure from homeostasis negatively impacts recovery and function, and ERAS protocols attempt to eliminate these problems.[4,5]

ENHANCED RECOVERY AFTER SURGERY: GENERAL PRINCIPLES

Medical centers around the world have been actively adopting protocols pioneered by Dr Kehlet and colleagues[1,2] dedicated to improving health care quality. They created a

Department of Anesthesiology and Critical Care, Perelman School of Medicine, University of Pennsylvania, 3400 Spruce Street, Dulles 680, Philadelphia, PA 19104, USA
* Corresponding author.
E-mail address: taras.grosh@uphs.upenn.edu

Anesthesiology Clin 36 (2018) 417–430
https://doi.org/10.1016/j.anclin.2018.04.006
1932-2275/18/© 2018 Elsevier Inc. All rights reserved.
anesthesiology.theclinics.com

structured clinical pathway for colorectal surgery and then reviewed its effectiveness after implementation. By auditing the outcome data for their pathway, Kehlet and colleagues[2] demonstrated a reduction in complications, hospital length of stay (LOS), and hospitalization cost. These pathways were designed to structure patient care with evidence-based interventions that improve perioperative experience and reduce unnecessary variations in care, time to discharge, and complications. The overarching goals of the colorectal ERAS protocol were to attenuate the physiologic disruptions from surgery through the use of goal-directed fluid therapy, modified bowel preparation, lung-protective ventilation, early mobilization, adequate warming, and multimodal analgesics and prophylaxis against postoperative nausea and vomiting (PONV).[6] Other goals include decreased morbidity and mortality,[7] decreased opioid consumption,[8] and increased patient satisfaction.[9] ERAS protocols are multidisciplinary in nature, encouraging collaboration among surgeons, anesthesiologists, nurses, physical therapists, and hospital administrators. Full commitment is needed from patients and providers, because lack of protocol adherence results in suboptimal management and failure to meet end points. **Fig. 1** illustrates how pathways are broken down into phases: preadmission, preoperative, intraoperative, and postoperative.

Given the success in colorectal surgery, other disciplines have adopted enhanced recovery protocols including gynecology, urology, and orthopedics. In knee and hip arthroplasty, clinical pathways focused around regional anesthesia and multimodal analgesia were superior to traditional general anesthesia (GA) and an opioid-centric model.[10] Hebl and colleagues[11] demonstrated the merits of a detailed protocol in the early 2000s for hip and knee arthroplasty. As early adopters, they reported decreases in total knee and hip arthroplasty hospital LOS and costs, especially in patients who have American Society of Anesthesiologists (ASA) physical status of 3 and above.[12] Moreover, the Mayo Clinic's Total Joint Regional Anesthesia Clinical Pathway states that the cornerstone to an effective protocol is peripheral nerve blockade and multimodal analgesia.[13]

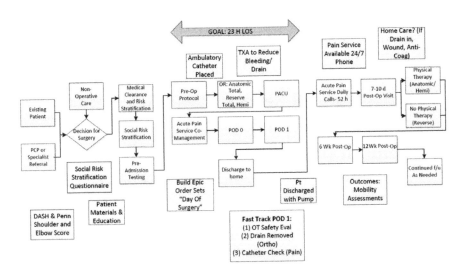

Fig. 1. Shoulder arthroplasty enhanced recovery protocol pathway. OR, operating room; OT, occupational therapy; PACU, postanesthesia care unit; PCP, primary care physician; POD, postop day; ShARP, Shoulder Arthroplasty enhanced Recovery Protocol; TXA, tranexamic acid.

To explore future health care delivery systems and payment models, the Center for Medicare and Medicaid Services created its Innovation Center, which introduced the Bundled Payments for Care Improvement initiative.[14] The first cohort started in 2013, and the goal of this initiative was to implement a single bundled payment for the multiple services beneficiaries receive during an episode of care. Under the initiative, organizations enter into payment arrangements that include financial and performance accountability for episodes of care.[14] The bundled payment model incentivizes hospitals to curb frivolous spending, reduce readmissions rates, eliminate complications, and deliver high-quality care by improving interdepartmental coordination while working with finite resources and staff. Hospitals and providers share the associated risk and financial penalties if they cannot control costs or if they fail to deliver quality health care.

In anticipation of these changes in health care, the ASA created the perioperative surgical home model.[15] The perioperative surgical home is a patient-centered, physician-led, interdisciplinary and team-based model, coordinating care from preprocedure assessment through the acute care episode, recovery, and postacute care. The goal is for each patient to receive the right care at the right place and at the right time, with the highest degree of satisfaction, fewer complications, and decreased costs. One essential component of the perioperative surgical home is establishment of procedure-specific ERAS protocols.

TOTAL SHOULDER ARTHROPLASTY

Shoulder arthroplasty has become the definitive treatment of painful end-stage shoulder glenohumeral osteoarthritis, rheumatoid arthritis, trauma, or osteonecrosis when conservative treatments have failed. In 2008, aa total of 47,000 procedures were performed in the United States[16]; that number is expected to increase dramatically because the demographics for shoulder arthroplasty are shifting to a younger population.[17,18] Depending on the pathology, multiple procedures exist: total shoulder arthroplasty, stemmed hemiarthroplasty, resurfacing hemiarthroplasty, and reverse total shoulder arthroplasty. These procedures are invasive but successful beyond 10 years in up to 90% of patients.[19] Afterward, patients can expect functional improvements that allow completion of their activities of daily living with a significant reduction, if not elimination, of preprocedural pain. For these patients, controlling immediate postoperative pain with opioids alone is a challenge, and prolonged hospital admission is expected if patients are unable to rehabilitate because of pain or experience opioid-related side effects. Beyond the commonly cited respiratory depression, constipation, pruritis, and nausea/vomiting seen in the immediate postoperative period, high-dose opioid dosing possesses its own set of complications in the form of tolerance, addiction, nociception-induced central sensitization,[20] and opioid-induced secondary hyperalgesia and persistent postsurgical pain.[21]

GENERAL VERSUS REGIONAL ANESTHESIA FOR TOTAL SHOULDER ARTHROPLASTY

Shoulder arthroplasty is performed under either general or regional anesthesia alone; most commonly a combination of GA and regional anesthesia is used.[22] Although GA is safe, convenient, and provides intraoperative amnesia, and akinesis, it has numerous side effects: nausea, vomiting, hoarseness, postoperative cognitive impairment, and potentially inadequate postoperative pain control. Each of these side effects or a combination of them can result in prolonged postanesthesia care unit stays and longer hospital admissions.[23] A retrospective study of 4158 patients found that regional anesthesia alone resulted in significantly greater rates of discharge to home versus institutionalized care, lower total in-hospital complications, and reduced rates of hospital readmission than GA.[24] In addition there were fewer unplanned readmissions for severe pain, sedation, and nausea/vomiting versus GA alone.[25] Unfortunately, regional anesthesia alone may not be appropriate routinely, because it requires an agreeable patient, a highly skilled surgeon comfortable with an awake/sedated patient, and an anesthesiologist who is proficient in regional anesthesia. Moreover, shoulder surgery can be prolonged with unpleasant stimuli, such as reaming of the humerus that, although not necessarily painful in the setting of an effective block, sometimes cannot be attenuated with sedation.[26] Furthermore, although having an awake patient reduces some concerns over inadequate cerebral oxygenation in the beach chair position, having limited access to an unsecured airway is challenging for the anesthesiologist.[27,28]

Regional anesthesia is still underused in the management of upper extremity surgeries and underimplemented in ERAS pathways.[29] Surgeons inappropriately cite increased risk of peripheral nerve injury,[30,31] the time it takes to perform, and inconsistent block results as reasons to avoid regional anesthesia.[32] The advent of ultrasound has allowed regional anesthesiologists to perform more consistent low-volume peripheral nerve blocks, which reduce the incidence of undesired side effects and even serious complications, such as local anesthetic systemic toxicity.[33] Additionally, ultrasound guidance has resulted in hastening the onset of nerve blocks and allowed precise perineural catheter placement for prolonged analgesia.[34] For shoulder surgeries, a variety of peripheral nerve blocks can target the brachial plexus and its branches: interscalene block (ISB), superior trunk block, or a combination of suprascapular[35] and axillary nerve blocks. Traditionally, an ISB targeting the C5 and C6 nerve roots provides adequate analgesia to much of the shoulder with a high likelihood of transient phrenic nerve palsy and hemidiaphragmatic involvement.[36] Superior trunk blocks target C5 and C6 more distally still capturing the suprascapular nerve but may spare the phrenic nerve. Additionally, because the suprascapular nerve provides 70% of sensation to the shoulder,[37] coupled with an axillary (circumflex) nerve block, patients reported 30% opioid reduction versus control and a reduction of nausea, vomiting, and LOS during shoulder arthroscopy.[35]

Unfortunately, the analgesic duration of a single injection block is limited by pharmacologic factors[38]; upper extremity blocks rarely exceed 18 hours even with adjuncts, such as clonidine, dexmedetomidine, or dexamethasone.[39] Higher concentration and/or volume of local anesthetic do not improve analgesia and instead may decrease patient satisfaction because of complete loss of motor function.[40] After single-injection blocks, patients are left vulnerable for rebound hyperalgesia[41] amplifying the worst of the acute postsurgical pain during the first 48 hours. For superior analgesia extending beyond the 48-hour "worst pain window," placement of a continuous perineural catheter is well supported in the literature[41–47]

Despite the success of ultrasound-guided procedures, perineural catheter placement is a complicated procedure with potentially serious complications.[48–50] Secondary catheter failure may result from catheter migration or initial misplacement that may be masked by bolusing the local anesthetic through the needle versus the catheter. Lastly, depending on the practice setting, some institutions may lack an acute pain service to do proper follow-up. Alternatively, surgeons may administer intra-articular and intramuscular injections of local anesthetic. More recently, liposomal bupivacaine has been introduced as an alternative longer duration local anesthetic. The evidence supporting local infiltration with liposomal bupivacaine is inconclusive.[51] A meta-analysis by Yan and coworkers[51] reviewed results from five studies (two randomized controlled trials, and three nonrandomized controlled trials, 573 patients, mainly small samples sizes), and found no statistical-significant differences in verbal analog scale (VAS) pain scores between the liposomal bupivacaine infiltration and ISB group at 4 hours, 8 hours, and 2 weeks. In addition, the liposomal bupivacaine group was associated with a reduction of VAS score of about 3 and 6 on a 100-point VAS scale at 12 and 24 hours. Finally, liposomal bupivacaine was associated with a reduction in hospital LOS by 0.16 days when compared with ISB; although statistically significant, this difference is unlikely to be clinically relevant. This analysis noted that many of the studies were underpowered, poorly designed, and industry sponsored. Generating additional concern is a literature review by Gulihar and colleagues[52] providing evidence that continuous periarticular and intra-articular injections are associated with chondrolysis.

ENHANCED RECOVERY AFTER SHOULDER SURGERY

Current protocols aim to improve patients' experience; deliver quality care; and reduce LOS, postoperative complications, and readmission rates. They are designed with a strong emphasis on improving postoperative pain management using regional anesthesia and multimodal analgesia.[53] Patient screening and optimization in the preoperative period are critical components of this protocol. Other components include PONV prophylaxis, use of antifibrinolytics,[54] and early involvement of occupational and physical therapy.

Herrick and colleagues[55] found that patients who have regional anesthesia as part of their anesthetic plan for shoulder arthroplasty had reduced rates of systemic complications, need for intensive care unit transfers, and prolonged hospital stay. Frederickson and colleagues[44] prospectively studied 1505 consecutive patients undergoing shoulder surgery (open and arthroscopic) who received continuous ISB at home and concluded that perineural catheters are safe and underused techniques for upper extremity surgery. Ilfeld and colleagues[56] demonstrated in a randomized placebo-controlled clinical trial that local anesthetic infusion through a perineural catheter decreased postoperative pain in shoulder arthroplasty patients by providing potent analgesia, increased patient satisfaction, decreased opioid requirements and their associated side effects, and decreased time to meet discharge eligibility. The results of this study emphasize the importance of continuous regional anesthesia in clinical pathways for shoulder surgery.

In 2014, YaDeau and colleagues[57] reported their institutional experience with a pilot clinical pathway specifically for shoulder arthroplasty using a single injection block approach supplemented with systemic nonopioid analgesics (ketamine, meloxicam, pregabalin, acetaminophen). They demonstrated opioid sparing, low pain scores, and high patient satisfaction. Ultimately, a single injection peripheral nerve block or perineural catheter is the greatest contributor to postoperative analgesia especially with movement by disrupting peripheral perception of surgical pain from reaching the central nervous system.

Given the ongoing opioid crisis, additional analgesic options are necessary. Clinical guidelines from ASA support acute care multimodal pain management recognizing the benefits of acetaminophen, nonsteroidal anti-inflammatory drugs,[58] gabapentinoids, and ketamine when combined with a peripheral nerve block and local infiltration[59] and encourage preventive analgesia.[60,61]

SHOULDER ARTHROPLASTY ENHANCED RECOVERY PROTOCOL

At the authors' institution (University of Pennsylvania), a Shoulder Arthroplasty enhanced Recovery Protocol (ShARP) was designed to improve patients' perioperative experience and outcomes. The protocol uses multimodal analgesia and features the use of regional anesthesia via a continuous ambulatory perineural catheter. It aims to decrease hospital LOS and complications after surgery. Since it started, it has been a resounding success with patients and health care providers.[55] We leveraged our prior experiences with implementation of a multimodal analgesia protocol in lower extremity joint arthroplasty and a home-based catheter program for outpatient shoulder arthroscopy. The main elements of ShARP are patient education, multimodal analgesia featuring ambulatory ISB, use of antifibrinolytic, and use of multimodal PONV prophylaxis. Common medications used for ERAS protocols are included in **Table 1**.

The first step in implementation of the protocol (see **Fig. 1**) was to invite all stakeholders (eg, surgeons, nurses, physical therapists, pharmacists) to discuss their individual perioperative goals and to learn their care processes. Second, we had to put together a vision for the pathway that accounts for each step of the patient's perioperative experience (see **Fig. 1**). We then had to circulate the draft of the pathway and revise it based on input from different stakeholders. Before we committed to the protocol, we proposed to pilot it for a trial period. Selection criteria for patients to be included in the ShARP were (1) availability of adequate home support, (2) a patient who is reliable and can take charge of own health, and (3) no major organ dysfunction.

A decision-making tool was built into the electronic medical record to answer yes or no to items 1 to 3 of the selection criteria listed previously. If the answer to each question is "yes," the patient is a ShARP candidate and flagged in the electronic medical record as such so all health care providers are alerted. If a patient did not meet all selection criteria, they would still go through the same ShARP care pathway but they were designated as non-ShARP. These patients would typically stay in the hospital for reasons related to their comorbidities or to socioeconomic issues that may have prevented earlier home discharge.

The pilot trial occurred extended between March and July 2016. We compared the LOS of total shoulder arthroplasty patients between March and July 2016 with a historical cohort of the same time frame (March to July) in 2015, which predated ShARP implementation. The initial results for the pilot trial were promising because we were able to reduce the average LOS from 3 days in 2015 to 1.5 days for all 2016 total shoulder arthroplasty patients (ShARP and non-ShARP) and down to 1.1 days for patients who were ShARP candidates.

Our conclusion is that putting in place some basic principles for better care will not only apply to patients who are good candidates to be in the protocol but will also lead to better outcomes for all patients. ShARP is now a mainstream practice in our institution and we are using it as a blueprint for designing and implementing other ERAS protocols in different surgical disciplines.

This experience has served to highlight the importance of the following key elements for successful implementation of ERAS protocols:

1. You have to define your outcome metrics a priori, often based on the type of surgery.
2. Collecting baseline data (before protocol implementation) is critical.
3. It is always recommended to start your protocol with a pilot trial within a given time period or defined by a predetermined number of patients.
4. Compare your baseline data against your pilot data to judge effectiveness and subsequently make a business plan for additional resources to expand your pathway.

Table 1
Common ERAS medications

	Name	Mechanism of Action	Dose	Comments
Nonopioid analgesics	Acetaminophen[62–64]	CNS: Inhibit COX-3, preventing formation and release of prostaglandins Periphery: Weak COX-1 and COX-2 inhibitor	Recommended dosing: 1000 mg q 6 h or 650 mg q 4 h Max single dose: 1000 mg Max daily dose: 4000 mg	Approved by the WHO as a treatment of mild to severe pain. Lacks the antiplatelet properties of NSAIDs and does not affect renal, cardiovascular, or gastric mucosa. IV acetaminophen leads to faster analgesic onset. Plasma concentrations peaks within 15 min. Its pharmacokinetics are more predictable than oral administration. Addition of IV acetaminophen to opioids resulted in reduced costs because of fewer adverse events and less time in the PACU. Use of IV vs oral formulation has to take cost effectiveness and patient ability to tolerate oral intake into account.

(continued on next page)

Table 1
(continued)

	Name	Mechanism of Action	Dose	Comments
Nonopioid analgesics	NSAIDs	Inhibit conversion of arachidonic acid to proinflammatory components in COX-2 pathway Inhibition of prostaglandin synthesis prevents activation of nociceptors; preventing peripheral tissue sensitization, secondary hyperalgesia, and minimizes central sensitization[65]	Propionic acid: Ibuprofen 400–800 mg q 4–8 h Max 2400 mg Naproxen 220 mg q 8 h Max 660 mg Coxib: Celecoxib 200 mg q 12 h Max 400 mg	COX-2 decreased opioid consumption and VAS pain score when compared with opioid alone or placebo after major orthopedic surgeries.[66,67] There are some concerns over increased risk of cardiovascular events[68] and delayed bone healing[69] with NSAID use.
	Antidepressants	Various mechanisms depending on type: TCA, SSRI, SNRI	Added to multimodal analgesia to decrease opioid consumption. Sufficient evidence is lacking for routine use of neuropathic pain medications for the prevention of chronic pain or for acute postoperative.[70] Large independent RCTs failed to demonstrate adequate analgesia during motion or opioid use reduction.[70]	
	Gabapentinoids	γ-Aminobutyric acid analogues bind to the α_2-delta receptors on voltage-gated calcium channels on presynaptic nerves Reduces the entry of calcium, decreasing the release of excitatory neurotransmitters (glutamate, aspartate, substance P, and norepinephrine) into the synaptic cleft Diminishes postsynaptic transmission of neural pain signals	Pregabalin 75 mg daily up to 600 mg daily Gabapentin 300 mg t.i.d. up to 3600 mg daily	Pregabalin: higher cost, but has a higher bioavailability allowing for more rapid titration. Gabapentinoids are anxiolytics,[71] improve sleep disturbance,[71] reduce the incidence of perioperative delirium,[72] and help prevent the onset of chronic postoperative pain.[73,74] Recent reports have brought to the attention the increased incidence of opioid side effects when mixed with gabapentinoids especially in elderly patients.[75]

Nonopioid analgesics	Ketamine	Noncompetitive *N*-methyl-D-aspartate receptor antagonist acts centrally in the dorsal horn of the spinal cord to decrease the release of glutamate and reduce transmission of pain messages centrally	IV bolus: 0.5 mg/kg followed by infusion: 0.15–0.25 mg/kg/h	It has opioid-sparing properties, reducing 24-h opioid requirements by 30%–50%, decreasing the incidence of opioid-related nausea and vomiting, improving analgesia,[76,77] and reducing the incidence of chronic pain.[78] Intravenous doses of 0.1–0.15 mg/kg ketamine improved early passive joint mobilization and hastened recovery in a group of patients having knee surgery.[77] Avidan et al[79] found that ketamine at doses of 0.5–1 mg/kg did not show evidence of reducing delirium, pain, or opioid consumption after surgery.
Antiemetics	Ondansetron, dexamethasone	Ondansetron is 5-HT3 receptor antagonist		Using multimodal PONV prophylaxis (5HT3, antihistamine, dopamine, anticholinergic, cannabinoid, corticosteroid) is superior to monotherapy. Evidence is lacking[80,81] that addition of dexamethasone is problematic to blood glucose in patients with diabetes. Dexamethasone offers an added benefit of the prolongation of a single injection peripheral nerve block[82] and prevents bupivacaine-induced rebound hyperalgesia.[83]
Antifibrinolytics	TXA	Competitively inhibits the activation of plasminogen to plasmin		TXA has shown a safe and significant reduction in perioperative blood loss and the requirement for allogeneic blood transfusion after TSA.[84,85] In our institutional experience, use of TXA in the setting of TSA has reduced the need for drain insertion and/or early removal of the drain on the first postoperative day; this has contributed to earlier hospital discharge.

A detailed review of medications used in ERAS pathways is beyond the scope of this article. This table is meant to give an overview of these medications.
Abbreviations: 5-HT3, 5-hydroxytryptamine; CNS, central nervous system; COX, cyclooxygenase enzyme; IV, intravenous; NSAIDs, nonsteroidal anti-inflammatory drugs; PACU, postanesthesia care unit; RCT, randomized controlled trial; SNRI, serotonin and norepinephrine reuptake inhibitors; SSRI, selective serotonin reuptake inhibitors; TCA, tricyclic antidepressants; TSA, total shoulder arthroplasty; TXA, tranexamic acid; WHO, World Health Organization.

REFERENCES

1. Ljungqvist O, Young-Fadok T, Demartines N. The history of enhanced recovery after surgery and the ERAS society. J Laparoendosc Adv Surg Tech A 2017; 27(9):860–2.
2. Tanious MK, Ljungqvist O, Urman RD. Enhanced recovery after surgery: history, evolution, guidelines, and future directions. Int Anesthesiol Clin 2017;55(4):1–11.
3. Haas DA, Kaplan RS. Variation in the cost of care for primary total knee arthroplasties. Arthroplast Today 2017;3(1):33–7.
4. Auyong DB, Allen CJ, Pahang JA, et al. Reduced length of hospitalization in primary total knee arthroplasty patients using an updated enhanced recovery after orthopedic surgery (ERAS) pathway. J Arthroplasty 2015;30(10):1705–9.
5. Ayalon O, Liu S, Flics S, et al. A multimodal clinical pathway can reduce length of stay after total knee arthroplasty. HSS J 2011;7(1):9–15.
6. Krenk L, Kehlet H, Baek Hansen T, et al. Cognitive dysfunction after fast-track hip and knee replacement. Anesth Analg 2014;118(5):1034–40.
7. Malviya A, Martin K, Harper I, et al. Enhanced recovery program for hip and knee replacement reduces death rate. Acta Orthop 2011;82(5):577–81.
8. Mathiesen O, Dahl B, Thomsen BA, et al. A comprehensive multimodal pain treatment reduces opioid consumption after multilevel spine surgery. Eur Spine J 2013;22(9):2089–96.
9. Gustafsson UO, Hausel J, Thorell A, et al. Adherence to the enhanced recovery after surgery protocol and outcomes after colorectal cancer surgery. Arch Surg 2011;146(5):571–7.
10. Barbieri A, Vanhaecht K, Van Herck P, et al. Effects of clinical pathways in the joint replacement: a meta-analysis. BMC Med 2009;7:32.
11. Hebl JR, Dilger JA, Byer DE, et al. A pre-emptive multimodal pathway featuring peripheral nerve block improves perioperative outcomes after major orthopedic surgery. Reg Anesth Pain Med 2008;33(6):510–7.
12. Horlocker TT, Kopp SL, Pagnano MW, et al. Analgesia for total hip and knee arthroplasty: a multimodal pathway featuring peripheral nerve block. J Am Acad Orthop Surg 2006;14(3):126–35.
13. Niesen AD, Hebl JR. Multimodal clinical pathways, perineural catheters, and ultrasound-guided regional anesthesia: the anesthesiologist's repertoire for the 21st century. Minn Med 2011;94(3):31–4.
14. Press MJ, Rajkumar R, Conway PH. Medicare's new bundled payments: design, strategy, and evolution. JAMA 2016;315(2):131–2.
15. Cannesson M, Kain Z. Enhanced recovery after surgery versus perioperative surgical home: is it all in the name? Anesth Analg 2014;118(5):901–2.
16. Day JS, Lau E, Ong KL, et al. Prevalence and projections of total shoulder and elbow arthroplasty in the United States to 2015. J Shoulder Elbow Surg 2010; 19(8):1115–20.
17. Kim SH, Wise BL, Zhang Y, et al. Increasing incidence of shoulder arthroplasty in the United States. J Bone Joint Surg Am 2011;93(24):2249–54.
18. Padegimas EM, Maltenfort M, Lazarus MD, et al. Future patient demand for shoulder arthroplasty by younger patients: national projections. Clin Orthop Relat Res 2015;473(6):1860–7.
19. Liu JN, Steinhaus ME, Garcia GH, et al. Return to sport after shoulder arthroplasty: a systematic review and meta-analysis. Knee Surg Sports Traumatol Arthrosc 2018;26(1):100–12.

20. Woolf CJ, Chong MS. Preemptive analgesia: treating postoperative pain by preventing the establishment of central sensitization. Anesth Analg 1993;77(2): 362–79.

21. Bjornholdt KT, Brandsborg B, Soballe K, et al. Persistent pain is common 1-2 years after shoulder replacement. Acta Orthop 2015;86(1):71–7.

22. Codding JL, Getz CL. Pain management strategies in shoulder arthroplasty. Orthop Clin North Am 2018;49(1):81–91.

23. Luo J, Min S. Postoperative pain management in the postanesthesia care unit: an update. J Pain Res 2017;10:2687–98.

24. Ding DY, Mahure SA, Mollon B, et al. Comparison of general versus isolated regional anesthesia in total shoulder arthroplasty: a retrospective propensity-matched cohort analysis. J Orthop 2017;14(4):417–24.

25. D'Alessio JG, Rosenblum M, Shea KP, et al. A retrospective comparison of inter-scalene block and general anesthesia for ambulatory surgery shoulder arthroscopy. Reg Anesth 1995;20(1):62–8.

26. Beecroft CL, Coventry DM. Anaesthesia for shoulder surgery. Continuing Education in Anaesthesia Critical Care & Pain 2008;8(6):193–8.

27. Aguirre JA, Marzendorfer O, Brada M, et al. Cerebral oxygenation in the beach chair position for shoulder surgery in regional anesthesia: impact on cerebral blood flow and neurobehavioral outcome. J Clin Anesth 2016;35:456–64.

28. Laflam A, Joshi B, Brady K, et al. Shoulder surgery in the beach chair position is associated with diminished cerebral autoregulation but no differences in postoperative cognition or brain injury biomarker levels compared with supine positioning: the anesthesia patient safety foundation beach chair study. Anesth Analg 2015;120(1):176–85.

29. Cozowicz C, Poeran J, Memtsoudis SG. Epidemiology, trends, and disparities in regional anaesthesia for orthopaedic surgery. Br J Anaesth 2015;115(Suppl 2): ii57–67.

30. Lupu CM, Kiehl TR, Chan VW, et al. Nerve expansion seen on ultrasound predicts histologic but not functional nerve injury after intraneural injection in pigs. Reg Anesth Pain Med 2010;35(2):132–9.

31. Sviggum HP, Jacob AK, Mantilla CB, et al. Perioperative nerve injury after total shoulder arthroplasty: assessment of risk after regional anesthesia. Reg Anesth Pain Med 2012;37(5):490–4.

32. Barrington MJ, Watts SA, Gledhill SR, et al. Preliminary results of the Australasian Regional Anaesthesia Collaboration: a prospective audit of more than 7000 peripheral nerve and plexus blocks for neurologic and other complications. Reg Anesth Pain Med 2009;34(6):534–41.

33. Barrington MJ, Kluger R. Ultrasound guidance reduces the risk of local anesthetic systemic toxicity following peripheral nerve blockade. Reg Anesth Pain Med 2013;38(4):289–99.

34. Mirza F, Brown AR. Ultrasound-guided regional anesthesia for procedures of the upper extremity. Anesthesiol Res Pract 2011;2011:579824.

35. Ritchie ED, Tong D, Chung F, et al. Suprascapular nerve block for postoperative pain relief in arthroscopic shoulder surgery: a new modality? Anesth Analg 1997; 84(6):1306–12.

36. Brown AR, Weiss R, Greenberg C, et al. Interscalene block for shoulder arthroscopy: comparison with general anesthesia. Arthroscopy 1993;9(3):295–300.

37. Neal JM, Gerancher JC, Hebl JR, et al. Upper extremity regional anesthesia: essentials of our current understanding, 2008. Reg Anesth Pain Med 2009;34(2): 134–70.

38. Fredrickson MJ, Krishnan S, Chen CY. Postoperative analgesia for shoulder surgery: a critical appraisal and review of current techniques. Anaesthesia 2010; 65(6):608–24.
39. Chong MA, Berbenetz NM, Lin C, et al. Perineural versus intravenous dexamethasone as an adjuvant for peripheral nerve blocks: a systematic review and meta-analysis. Reg Anesth Pain Med 2017;42(3):319–26.
40. Fredrickson MJ, Smith KR, Wong AC. Importance of volume and concentration for ropivacaine interscalene block in preventing recovery room pain and minimizing motor block after shoulder surgery. Anesthesiology 2010;112(6):1374–81.
41. Fredrickson MJ, Ball CM, Dalgleish AJ. Analgesic effectiveness of a continuous versus single-injection interscalene block for minor arthroscopic shoulder surgery. Reg Anesth Pain Med 2010;35(1):28–33.
42. Baskan S, Cankaya D, Unal H, et al. Comparison of continuous interscalene block and subacromial infusion of local anesthetic for postoperative analgesia after open shoulder surgery. J Orthop Surg (Hong Kong) 2017;25(1). 2309499016684093.
43. Chidiac EJ, Kaddoum R, Peterson SA. Patient survey of continuous interscalene analgesia at home after shoulder surgery. Middle East J Anaesthesiol 2009;20(2): 213–8.
44. Fredrickson MJ, Leightley P, Wong A, et al. An analysis of 1505 consecutive patients receiving continuous interscalene analgesia at home: a multicentre prospective safety study. Anaesthesia 2016;71(4):373–9.
45. Ullah H, Samad K, Khan FA. Continuous interscalene brachial plexus block versus parenteral analgesia for postoperative pain relief after major shoulder surgery. Cochrane Database Syst Rev 2014;(2):CD007080.
46. Ilfeld BM, Morey TE, Wright TW, et al. Continuous interscalene brachial plexus block for postoperative pain control at home: a randomized, double-blinded, placebo-controlled study. Anesth Analg 2003;96(4):1089–95. Table of contents.
47. Mariano ER, Afra R, Loland VJ, et al. Continuous interscalene brachial plexus block via an ultrasound-guided posterior approach: a randomized, triple-masked, placebo-controlled study. Anesth Analg 2009;108(5):1688–94.
48. Boezaart AP, Tighe P. New trends in regional anesthesia for shoulder surgery: avoiding devastating complications. Int J Shoulder Surg 2010;4(1):1–7.
49. Capdevila X, Jaber S, Pesonen P, et al. Acute neck cellulitis and mediastinitis complicating a continuous interscalene block. Anesth Analg 2008;107(4): 1419–21.
50. Yanovski B, Gaitini L, Volodarski D, et al. Catastrophic complication of an interscalene catheter for continuous peripheral nerve block analgesia. Anaesthesia 2012;67(10):1166–9.
51. Yan Z, Chen Z, Ma C. Liposomal bupivacaine versus interscalene nerve block for pain control after shoulder arthroplasty: a meta-analysis. Medicine (Baltimore) 2017;96(27):e7226.
52. Gulihar A, Robati S, Twaij H, et al. Articular cartilage and local anaesthetic: A systematic review of the current literature. J Orthop 2015;12(Suppl 2):S200-10.
53. Warrender WJ, Syed UAM, Hammoud S, et al. Pain management after outpatient shoulder arthroscopy: a systematic review of randomized controlled trials. Am J Sports Med 2017;45(7):1676–86.
54. Soffin EM, YaDeau JT. Enhanced recovery after surgery for primary hip and knee arthroplasty: a review of the evidence. Br J Anaesth 2016;117(suppl 3):iii62–72.

55. Herrick MD, Liu H, Davis M, et al. Regional anesthesia decreases complications and resource utilization in shoulder arthroplasty patients. Acta Anaesthesiol Scand 2018;62(4):540–7.
56. Ilfeld BM, Vandenborne K, Duncan PW, et al. Ambulatory continuous interscalene nerve blocks decrease the time to discharge readiness after total shoulder arthroplasty: a randomized, triple-masked, placebo-controlled study. Anesthesiology 2006;105(5):999–1007.
57. Goon AK, Dines DM, Craig EV, et al. A clinical pathway for total shoulder arthroplasty: a pilot study. HSS J 2014;10(2):100–6.
58. Pavlin DJ, Chen C, Penaloza DA, et al. Pain as a factor complicating recovery and discharge after ambulatory surgery. Anesth Analg 2002;95(3):627–34. Table of contents.
59. American Society of Anesthesiologists Task Force on Acute Pain Management. Practice guidelines for acute pain management in the perioperative setting: an updated report by the American Society of Anesthesiologists Task Force on Acute Pain Management. Anesthesiology 2012;116(2):248–73.
60. Diaz-Heredia J, Loza E, Cebreiro I, et al. Preventive analgesia in hip or knee arthroplasty: a systematic review. Rev Esp Cir Ortop Traumatol 2015;59(2):73–90.
61. Tang R, Evans H, Chaput A, et al. Multimodal analgesia for hip arthroplasty. Orthop Clin North Am 2009;40(3):377–87.
62. Singla NK, Parulan C, Samson R, et al. Plasma and cerebrospinal fluid pharmacokinetic parameters after single-dose administration of intravenous, oral, or rectal acetaminophen. Pain Pract 2012;12(7):523–32.
63. Subramanyam R, Varughese A, Kurth CD, et al. Cost-effectiveness of intravenous acetaminophen for pediatric tonsillectomy. Paediatr Anaesth 2014;24(5):467–75.
64. Apfel CC, Turan A, Souza K, et al. Intravenous acetaminophen reduces postoperative nausea and vomiting: a systematic review and meta-analysis. Pain 2013; 154(5):677–89.
65. Katz WA. Cyclooxygenase-2-selective inhibitors in the management of acute and perioperative pain. Cleve Clin J Med 2002;69(Suppl 1):SI65–75.
66. Buvanendran A, Kroin JS, Tuman KJ, et al. Effects of perioperative administration of a selective cyclooxygenase 2 inhibitor on pain management and recovery of function after knee replacement: a randomized controlled trial. JAMA 2003; 290(18):2411–8.
67. Diaz-Borjon E, Torres-Gomez A, Essex MN, et al. Parecoxib provides analgesic and opioid-sparing effects following major orthopedic surgery: a subset analysis of a randomized, placebo-controlled clinical trial. Pain Ther 2017;6(1):61–72.
68. Nussmeier NA, Whelton AA, Brown MT, et al. Safety and efficacy of the cyclooxygenase-2 inhibitors parecoxib and valdecoxib after noncardiac surgery. Anesthesiology 2006;104(3):518–26.
69. Marquez-Lara A, Hutchinson ID, Nuñez F Jr, et al. Nonsteroidal anti-inflammatory drugs and bone-healing: a systematic review of research quality. JBJS Rev 2016; 4(3) [pii:01874474-201603000-00005].
70. Mathiesen O, Wetterslev J, Kontinen VK, et al. Adverse effects of perioperative paracetamol, NSAIDs, glucocorticoids, gabapentinoids and their combinations: a topical review. Acta Anaesthesiol Scand 2014;58(10):1182–98.
71. Sabatowski R, Galvez R, Cherry DA, et al. Pregabalin reduces pain and improves sleep and mood disturbances in patients with post-herpetic neuralgia: results of a randomised, placebo-controlled clinical trial. Pain 2004;109(1–2):26–35.
72. Leung JM, Sands LP, Rico M, et al. Pilot clinical trial of gabapentin to decrease postoperative delirium in older patients. Neurology 2006;67(7):1251–3.

73. Clarke H, Bonin RP, Orser BA, et al. The prevention of chronic postsurgical pain using gabapentin and pregabalin: a combined systematic review and meta-analysis. Anesth Analg 2012;115(2):428–42.
74. Sawan H, Chen AF, Viscusi ER, et al. Pregabalin reduces opioid consumption and improves outcome in chronic pain patients undergoing total knee arthroplasty. Phys Sportsmed 2014;42(2):10–8.
75. Gomes T, Juurlink DN, Antoniou T, et al. Gabapentin, opioids, and the risk of opioid-related death: a population-based nested case–control study. PLOS Med 2017;14(10):e1002396.
76. Jouguelet-Lacoste J, La Colla L, Schilling D, et al. The use of intravenous infusion or single dose of low-dose ketamine for postoperative analgesia: a review of the current literature. Pain Med 2015;16(2):383–403.
77. Menigaux C, Fletcher D, Dupont X, et al. The benefits of intraoperative small-dose ketamine on postoperative pain after anterior cruciate ligament repair. Anesth Analg 2000;90(1):129–35.
78. Remerand F, Le Tendre C, Baud A, et al. The early and delayed analgesic effects of ketamine after total hip arthroplasty: a prospective, randomized, controlled, double-blind study. Anesth Analg 2009;109(6):1963–71.
79. Avidan MS, Maybrier HR, Abdallah AB, et al. Intraoperative ketamine for prevention of postoperative delirium or pain after major surgery in older adults: an international, multicentre, double-blind, randomised clinical trial. Lancet 2017; 390(10091):267–75.
80. Nurok M, Cheng J, Romeo GR, et al. Dexamethasone and perioperative blood glucose in patients undergoing total joint arthroplasty: a retrospective study. J Clin Anesth 2017;37:116–22.
81. De Oliveira GS Jr, Castro-Alves LJ, Ahmad S, et al. Dexamethasone to prevent postoperative nausea and vomiting: an updated meta-analysis of randomized controlled trials. Anesth Analg 2013;116(1):58–74.
82. Zhao WL, Ou XF, Liu J, et al. Perineural versus intravenous dexamethasone as an adjuvant in regional anesthesia: a systematic review and meta-analysis. J Pain Res 2017;10:1529–43.
83. An K, Elkassabany NM, Liu J. Dexamethasone as adjuvant to bupivacaine prolongs the duration of thermal antinociception and prevents bupivacaine-induced rebound hyperalgesia via regional mechanism in a mouse sciatic nerve block model. PLoS One 2015;10(4):e0123459.
84. Gillespie R, Shishani Y, Joseph S, et al. A randomized, prospective evaluation on the effectiveness of tranexamic acid in reducing blood loss after total shoulder arthroplasty. J Shoulder Elbow Surg 2015;24:1679–84.
85. Friedman R, Gordon E, Butler R, et al. Tranexamic acid decreases blood loss after total shoulder arthroplasty. J Shoulder Elbow Surg 2016;25:614–8.

Regional Anesthesia and Analgesia for Acute Trauma Patients

Ian R. Slade, MD[a],*, Ron E. Samet, MD[b]

KEYWORDS

- Trauma • Trauma pain • Trauma analgesia • Regional anesthesia
- Peripheral nerve block • Neuraxial block

KEY POINTS

- Compared with traditional analgesic modalities, peripheral nerve blockade (PNB) provides trauma patients with superior pain relief targeted to the site(s) of injury.
- PNB use in trauma may decrease morbidity and mortality, promote favorable surgical outcomes, and decrease length of stay in some circumstances.
- PNB skills are increasingly being taught to prehospital and emergency medicine providers with direct benefit to acute trauma patients.
- PNB decreases acute opioid use, avoiding related side effects, important for patient safety and comfort.
- Although data are scarce, early PNB may reduce the incidence or severity of chronic pain and subsequent opioid use, a consideration in the present opioid epidemic.

INTRODUCTION

The role of regional anesthesia in trauma care has grown substantially over the past few decades. Rapid advancements in techniques involving high-fidelity ultrasound and an ensuing proliferation of educational materials have made learning peripheral nerve blockade (PNB) more accessible. Since the first description of an ulnar nerve block with cocaine to enable the pain-free removal of a bullet by Burke[1] in 1884, a multitude of nerve block procedures were developed to provide analgesia and surgical anesthesia for most regions of the body by the mid-twentieth century, although these methods were not developed specifically for use in trauma.[2]

Disclosure Statement: The authors have nothing to disclose.
[a] Department of Anesthesiology and Pain Medicine, Harborview Medical Center, University of Washington School of Medicine, 325 9th Avenue, Box 359724, Seattle, WA 98104, USA; [b] Department of Anesthesiology, Division of Trauma Anesthesiology, R Adams Cowley Shock Trauma Center, University of Maryland Medical Center, University of Maryland School of Medicine, 22 South Greene Street, Baltimore, MD 21201, USA
* Corresponding author.
E-mail address: islade@u.washington.edu

Anesthesiology Clin 36 (2018) 431–454
https://doi.org/10.1016/j.anclin.2018.04.004
1932-2275/18/© 2018 Elsevier Inc. All rights reserved.

anesthesiology.theclinics.com

Military trauma care units, in particular, used PNB to deliver targeted limb analgesia and enable surgical interventions in resource-scarce environments, often while preserving airway patency, mental status, and hemodynamics. The superior stability and patient comfort permitted easier evacuation of wounded patients to higher levels of care.[3] However, with perineural local anesthetic injection came the rare but potentially catastrophic risk of local anesthetic systemic toxicity (LAST) and postblock neurologic injuries, resulting in more limited use and the need to develop safer medications and methods of administration.[2] Since the 1970s, new techniques and ultrasound guidance have reinvigorated the role PNB plays in perioperative care by anesthesia teams. This expertise has extended to combat and civilian trauma management, with prehospital providers, advanced nurse practitioners, and physicians in the emergency department (ED) beginning to offer these techniques in certain situations, as well.[4–10]

When practicing regional anesthesia in trauma care, advantages and indications beyond acute analgesia have been discovered that warrant further investigation and validation in this patient population. Likewise, unique concerns and considerations have emerged that differentiate PNB application in the acutely injured patient from the elective surgical patient. There remains great potential for clinical research to delineate indications, optimal techniques, and outcomes for use of PNB in trauma. This article reviews the current literature and discusses future directions of regional anesthesia in the acute trauma patient.

ADVANTAGES OF REGIONAL ANESTHETIC TECHNIQUES

The most recognized indication and advantage of regional anesthesia in trauma patients is the provision of acute pain relief and/or dense anesthesia to a specific injured area of the body. Rapid and sometimes complete pain relief achieved via regional block provides compassionate analgesia and is reported to be more effective than traditional approaches using systemic opioids and sedatives.[11,12] However, there are additional secondary advantages and indications in the trauma population that require more attention and are the focus of ongoing research.

PERIPHERAL NERVE BLOCKS

Despite a lack of robust outcome data, trauma teams are expanding use of PNB techniques, believing that the benefits of selected blocks outweigh risks of systemic analgesics for certain patients. As safe, teachable, and generally reproducible interventions that require little time to perform, PNB can provide excellent analgesia without disruptions in hemodynamics or respiratory status. Other benefits include less opioid intake with reduced opioid-related side effects and sedation, permitting better assessment of mental status changes and acute surgical conditions. Long-term effects from early nerve blockade may include reduction in the incidence and severity of chronic posttraumatic pain syndromes,[13,14] better surgical outcomes with immobilization of delicate neurovascular repairs,[15] and greater tolerance of aggressive physical therapy.[16] Sympathetic inhibition and decreased catecholamine release from PNB have the potential to improve vascular flow and decrease vasospasm.[17] In austere environments, regional anesthesia allows for quicker triage, earlier readiness for transport, and reduced costs compared with general anesthesia and systemic medications. Finally, perhaps most importantly, PNB seems promising to decrease morbidity and mortality when patients are at increased risk of aspiration, present a difficult airway (with or without a cervical collar), or have multiple comorbid diseases that stratify them at higher risk of complications from general anesthesia or deep sedation. Unfortunately, many of these additional benefits and indications have yet to be proven in large outcome studies, perhaps leading to underutilization of PNB by many trauma practitioners to date.

NEURAXIAL BLOCK

Before the proliferation of PNB, neuraxial blockade was the primary regional analgesic for thoracic, abdominal, and lower extremity trauma. Spinal blockade allowed for dense rapid anesthesia with preservation of the awake state, and continuous epidural block provided long-lasting analgesia for painful injuries. However, catastrophic block-related complications owing to traumatic hypovolemia and hemodynamic instability, coagulopathy, neurologic deficit, or elevated intracranial pressure precluded universal application. Furthermore, insertion and management of neuraxial techniques requires appropriately experienced providers, special patient positioning, greater monitoring, and time, usually relegating these techniques to in-hospital anesthesiology services. With the need for thromboprophylaxis in recumbent trauma patients or therapeutic anticoagulation after vascular injuries, the trauma team must carefully coordinate initiation and discontinuation of neuraxial blocks to reduce risk for complications. Due to the multifactorial concerns, a more cautious risk/benefit analysis regarding administration of neuraxial anesthesia should be conducted with consideration of peripheral nerve and interfascial plane blocks as alternative options, depending on the indications.

Interestingly, the Eastern Association for the Surgery of Trauma (EAST) practice management guidelines workgroup in 2005 designated thoracic epidural analgesia as a level I recommendation for pain management after rib fractures.[18] However, recent studies have challenged their utility and point to possible harm. McKendy and colleagues[19] found increased respiratory complications and hospital length of stay (LOS) in 240 blunt trauma patients with more than 1 fractured rib who were treated with epidural analgesia compared with a nonepidural cohort. Similarly, a 10-year retrospective review at a level 1 trauma center found epidural catheter placement to be associated with increased rates of deep vein thrombosis, an increase in hospital LOS, yet decreased mortality.[20] Options for truncal analgesia have expanded beyond neuraxial approaches thanks to innovative, more peripheral techniques, such as ultrasound-guided paravertebral, transversus abdominis plane, intercostal, serratus anterior plane, and erector spinae plane blocks.[21–26] For example, Bossolasco and colleagues[21] achieved dramatic analgesia and resolution of respiratory splinting in an obese motor vehicle accident victim who suffered unilateral fractures of the second through ninth ribs using a continuous serratus anterior muscle plane block, whereas Hamilton and Manickam[23] produced similar effects from a continuous erector spinae plane block for multiple traumatic unilateral rib fractures in an acute thoracic trauma patient.

With inconclusive data for epidural analgesia, these newer techniques hold promise for offering similar analgesic efficacy with significantly fewer side effects and contraindications, and are gaining popularity as first-line treatments. In this light, EAST and the Trauma Anesthesiology Society have modified their expert consensus on epidural analgesia to a "conditional" recommendation[27] as improvements in duration of mechanical ventilation, intensive care unit or hospital LOS, or mortality have not been demonstrated in a large meta-analysis.[28] Further research to clarify optimal analgesic strategies for rib fracture management will inform trauma systems in developing comprehensive multiple rib fracture protocols based on injury severity, location, and morbidity.

CURRENT TRENDS IN REGIONAL ANALGESIA FOR TRAUMA

Historically, regional anesthesia techniques were in-hospital procedures used for perioperative anesthesia or analgesia almost exclusively by physician anesthesiologists. Fortunately for acute trauma patients, this trend is shifting. As regional anesthesia experience expands, prehospital providers, emergency medicine practitioners, and nurse-led services in some settings have begun to offer PNB to patients. A summary of these trends is presented in **Table 1**.

PREHOSPITAL

As noted in the introduction, military use of prehospital regional block techniques is well described.[3,29] In some civilian locales where physicians are part of the prehospital response team, on-scene PNB can achieve rapid analgesia in injured patients. For example, in France, anesthesia-trained prehospital providers have published reports of acute trauma victims benefiting from femoral,[5] fascia iliaca,[7,8] sciatic,[30] and interscalene[31] PNB. In 2 of these studies, paramedics or emergency medical service nurses were trained to perform fascia iliaca compartment blocks to significantly reduce pain scores from femur fractures and allow for more comfortable hospital transfer.[7,8]

Case reports from the military describe the safe and comfortable transport of injured soldiers with PNB catheters from initial triage units to definitive care facilities. Civilian trauma centers have followed suit with outpatient continuous PNB, especially when discharging to acute rehabilitation facilities that are familiar with these devices.[32]

EMERGENCY DEPARTMENT

With "oligoanalgesia" quite common among adult and pediatric trauma patients in prehospital and emergency medicine,[33–35] many efforts are focused on bettering trauma pain management.[36] The Centers for Medicare and Medicaid Services developed a quality measure for the time it takes patients with long-bone fracture to receive pain medication after arriving in the ED.[37] The Joint Commission Comprehensive Accreditation Manual for Hospitals is stressing early pain management for trauma patients.[38] Challenges in meeting adequate analgesic goals are exacerbated in the wake of the current opioid epidemic[39] and in the large proportion of substance abuse trauma patients in whom standard intravenous medications are unsatisfactory.[40,41] The need to appropriately tackle acute trauma pain with alternative modalities has grown and requires a new approach.[42]

Inspired by the ease and safety of newly described ultrasound-guided regional anesthesia techniques in perioperative medicine, early emergency medicine adopters began to realize the benefits of PNB in their patient population.[43] Blaivas and colleagues[12] reported excellent analgesia, avoiding intravenous sedation, after interscalene blocks in the ED for treating shoulder dislocation, and Stewart and colleagues[44] obtained superb analgesia by continuous femoral nerve block catheters in children with femur fractures in the ED. A proliferation of more recent studies from emergency medicine report similar results,[45–47] leading some to advocate for more universal training of regional anesthesia in emergency medicine curricula and training programs.[4] Secondary benefits of decreased monitoring, fewer side effects from systemic analgesics, and shorter lengths of stay by several hours when comparing supraclavicular brachial plexus block versus procedural sedation in upper extremity injuries[48] has garnered additional interest in busy and resource-limited EDs. With ultrasound diagnostics rapidly expanding in acute trauma care (eg, extended focused

Table 1
Summary of current trends in regional anesthesia for trauma

Primary Objectives	Provider Groups	PNB Techniques Reported	Challenges
Prehospital			
• Early analgesia • Decrease need for opioids and sedatives • Facilitate smooth transport to hospital	• Paramedics • EMS nurses • Prehospital physicians	• Interscalene • Femoral • Fascia iliaca • Sciatic	• Diagnostic accuracy of injury and thorough neurologic examination before block • Appropriateness of patient selection • Consistency of training, experience, and oversight • Preparedness for recognizing and treating LAST • Limited opportunity for ultrasound guidance • Time needed to perform block vs urgency of transport
ED			
• Earlier pain relief addresses concerns of oligoanalgesia in trauma care • Decrease need for opioids and sedatives • Provide superior analgesia, likely to be effective even in opioid-tolerant patients • Preserve consciousness and airway protection • Reduce pain from distracting injury and enable further assessment of concurrent injuries • Avoid deep sedation for ED procedures and the need for close monitoring during sedation recovery (and shorten ED length of stay)	• Anesthesiologists • CRNAs • Emergency medicine physicians • Advanced practice nurses	• Most of the common PNB techniques for upper and lower extremities • Non-neuraxial truncal blocks • Neuraxial block (sparingly)	• Prioritization of primary survey and early resuscitation • Consistency of training, experience, and oversight • Preparedness for recognizing and treating LAST • Availability of equipment, space, and time • Satisfactory patient positioning

(continued on next page)

Table 1
(continued)

Perioperative

Primary Objectives	Provider Groups	PNB Techniques Reported	Challenges
• Can avoid airway and hemodynamic consequences of deep sedation or general anesthesia • Facilitate positioning (eg, femoral block before performing spinal anesthesia for femur fracture) • Continuous PNB can facilitate repeated painful procedures (wound care) • Decreased reliance on opioids and their side effects • Improved comfort promotes greater mobility and participation in rehabilitative therapies • Improve blood flow to injured extremity • May protect fresh neurovascular or tendon repairs • Possibly decrease long-term opioid use and tolerance or abuse • Possible impact on development of chronic pain	• Anesthesiologists • CRNAs	• All PNB techniques for upper and lower extremities • Non-neuraxial truncal blocks (paravertebral, erector spinae plane, serratus anterior plane, transversus abdominis plane, rectus abdominis plane, quadratus lumborum) • Neuraxial block	• If PNB is intended as primary anesthetic, must be prepared for block failure and need for rapid GA conversion • Continuous PNB placement may interfere with surgical approach

Abbreviations: CRNA, certified registered nurse anesthetist; ED, emergency department; EMS, emergency medical services; GA, general anesthesia; LAST, local anesthetic systemic toxicity; PNB, peripheral nerve block.

assessment with sonography for trauma [E-FAST] examinations, transcranial ultrasound, fracture determination), and as more non–anesthesiology-trained providers use this technology, continued growth of PNB is likely to occur in the ED setting.

PERIOPERATIVE

Undoubtedly, the bulk of experience with regional block techniques originated in anesthesiology, where PNBs have long been an integral component of perioperative management. As sole anesthetics or part of a multimodal approach to analgesia, nerve blocks have touted superb pain relief and a better side-effect profile compared with sedation and general anesthesia. For example, brachial plexus block for upper extremity injuries or femoral and sciatic nerve blocks for lower extremity trauma are routinely used in isolated limb trauma surgery with some patients avoiding systemic anesthetics altogether.[49] When serial debridements or frequent painful wound care and dressing changes are needed, perineural catheters are often requested to alleviate the need for potent opioids, deep sedation, or general anesthesia.[50] In truncal and abdominal trauma as well, novel ultrasound-guided interfascial plane blocks are demonstrating effective pain relief.

PNB also can provide important indirect benefits in these patients. For example, administering a femoral nerve block or fascia iliaca block to facilitate placement of spinal anesthesia for patients with femur fracture demonstrated lower pain scores and better positioning for neuraxial block when compared with intravenous opioids in 2 studies.[51,52] When considering the incidence and severity of chronic pain syndromes after trauma, such as complex regional pain syndrome or phantom limb pain (PLP), studies have shown that early nerve blockade may significantly reduce challenging pain symptoms months to years after the injury.[13,14] A case series of 10 trauma patients with upper limb amputation reported reduced intensity of PLP symptoms after a continuous brachial plexus PNB and memantine was provided.[53] Additional studies with larger cohorts are needed to more definitively value the role of both early and late PNB in mediating symptoms of chronic pain after trauma.

Any intervention that can improve surgical outcomes and decrease perioperative morbidity and mortality demands investigation and strong consideration. Despite no published evidence that PNB improves the chances of long-term tissue viability or function in trauma surgery, trauma teams and anesthesiologists extrapolate from higher rates of graft and fistula patency reported in microvascular and arteriovenous fistula creation surgery[54] to suggest PNB can enhance blood flow to injured tissue, both via a regional sympathectomy and by improved pain relief decreasing catecholamine release. Other advantages may include preventing undesired movements of freshly repaired structures via a motor block, and providing analgesia to facilitate better tolerance of physical therapy.[15,16]

Although the overall safety of general anesthesia has markedly improved over the past several decades, there may be compelling reasons to avoid it in acutely compromised trauma patients. Sedation, general anesthesia, and endotracheal intubation all carry greater risk in patients with hypovolemia, full stomachs, and potentially compromised airway access due to cervical spine mobility precautions. The respiratory depression, nausea and vomiting, pruritus, and hemodynamic effects of opioids interfere with the immediate safety, comfort, and frequent mental status assessments vital to trauma care. When PNB can alleviate distracting pain and preserve consciousness, patients may participate in secondary and tertiary trauma surveys, thereby expediting evaluation of injuries and prioritizing care. Last, in the present opioid epidemic, multimodal analgesia, including PNB, may reduce opioid needs sufficiently for some patients to decrease risk of chronic use.[42]

SPECIAL CONSIDERATIONS IN TRAUMA

Despite PNB's many advantages, acute trauma patients present a unique set of challenges compared with elective surgical patients (**Table 2**). For example, the presence of brain injury, emotional distress, distracting painful injuries, chemical impairment, hemodynamic instability, and coagulopathy are common in the polytrauma patient. Such conditions may alter patients' ability to participate in decision-making, safely cooperate with block placement, or allow providers to properly assess for block efficacy and potential complications. Refer to **Table 3** for a full listing of special considerations by specific block technique.

INFORMED CONSENT

Obtaining informed consent may be difficult or even impossible in the presence of the distress accompanying acute trauma. Even patients who are conscious and communicative may have life-threatening injuries that require emergent management, without time for a detailed discussion of indications, risks, benefits, and alternatives of proposed interventions with them or their surrogate. Some treatments can be ethically justified under the principles of implied consent when there is immediate threat to life, limb, or vision. Although PNB is generally safe and improves patient comfort, it is frequently considered an elective intervention. However, in some circumstances, alternate modes of analgesia and anxiolysis may have greater likelihood of causing harm. For example, performing targeted PNB for emergent fracture reduction to preserve limb/tissue viability may offer less risk than possible airway or hemodynamic compromise resulting from deep sedation or general anesthesia in a full-stomach trauma patient. Institution-based protocols regarding surrogate consent or implied consent should be followed, with documented justification for the particular PNB intervention in the emergent setting.

BLOCKS AND IMPAIRED CONSCIOUSNESS

The relative safety of placing blocks in awake patients compared with those who are sedated, anesthetized, or who have impaired consciousness from brain injury or intoxication remains an area of controversy. The American Society of Regional Anesthesia (ASRA) guidelines continue to advocate for the performance of regional anesthetics in awake or sedated patients while maintaining meaningful contact in cooperative adult patients,[55] with particular concern for interscalene or neuraxial procedures after case reports posit a heightened association between postblock nerve injuries and the unresponsive state of a patient at the time of the block.[56–58] Others argue, however, that, when indicated, an anesthetized patient may provide more optimal conditions to allow for a more controlled and safe targeted technique.[59] Regional blocks in the "asleep" pediatric population are well-established with a recent analysis of more than 50,000 patients from the Pediatric Regional Anesthesia Network supporting the safety of placing both neuraxial and PNB in anesthetized children.[60] Anecdotally, the authors consider acute adult trauma patients to have potential indications and advantages for asleep blocks when excessive pain, decreased mental status, or optimal timing of the regional block preclude performance in the awake, responsive state. With appropriate informed consent, as discussed previously, performance of neuraxial or

Table 2
Summary of special considerations in trauma

Topic	Challenges	Potential Approaches
Consent	• Impaired consciousness • Judgment impaired by psychiatric condition, substance use, or iatrogenic medicines • Acute distress impairs comprehension and capacity for voluntary agreement, threatening validity of consent • Life-threatening conditions take priority; insufficient time for consent discussion with patient/surrogate • PNB usually seen as elective, nonessential intervention	• If PNB benefits seem highly likely to outweigh risks of alternative methods, seek informed consent from surrogate (and assent from patient, when possible) • If patient requires an urgent procedure for a condition that threatens life or limb, and sedation and/or opioids present an added risk of complications, may be able to ethically justify PNB as suitable alternative
Impaired consciousness	• Common in trauma patient due to intoxication, brain injury, shock state, or need for sedation or general anesthesia in acute injury • Controversy about heightened risk of nerve injury in "asleep" patient	• Ultrasound may theoretically avoid needle-to-nerve contact if desired • Consider fascial plane blocks, when indicated, to avoid direct neural contact
Prioritizing resuscitation	• Critical to act quickly to preserve life and prevent secondary injury • ATLS protocols vital for organized and comprehensive assessment; may not have flexibility to permit time for safe regional anesthetic • Impaired consciousness complicates assessment of block safety and efficacy	• Work with trauma team to complete necessary steps of primary and secondary survey • Participate in shared decision-making about risks, benefits, and alternatives of pain management strategies, and consider if/when regional analgesia may have a role
Positioning limitations	• Most trauma patients need to be supine for assessment, treatment, and maintaining safe hemodynamics • Neuraxial blocks and PNB requiring posterior approach may not be feasible • Injury may make certain positioning intolerably painful • Cervical collar may interfere with access for some upper extremity blocks	• Ultrasound permits ready visualization of targets for PNB in many regions of the body without needing repositioning • For injury to trunk, consider peripheral truncal blocks rather than neuraxial or paraneuraxial approach • Prudent to set up all regional equipment before positioning patient

(continued on next page)

Table 2
(continued)

Topic	Challenges	Potential Approaches
Coagulopathy	• Acquired coagulopathy is present in many trauma patients • Unknown medical history and whether patient is chronically coagulopathic • Effects of newer anticoagulant drugs may not be evident from routine blood testing • Bleeding consequences from neuraxial block may cause paralysis • Life-threatening hemorrhage possible if undetected bleeding in deep blocks • Paucity of evidence regarding safety of PNB in the presence of varying anticoagulant/antiplatelet drugs/doses • Unclear whether provider experience or ultrasound use alters bleeding risk	• Avoid neuraxial and paraneuraxial procedures in acute trauma until sufficient information known about coagulation status and medical history • Have informed discussion with patient or surrogate when considering PNB in the presence of any coagulopathy • If PNB still seems strongly indicated over alternatives, may consider superficial PNB in regions that are compressible should bleeding occur • Discuss DVT prophylaxis and any plans for therapeutic anticoagulation with trauma team to coordinate block initiation and discontinuation
Nerve injury	• Acute nerve injury may be present in acute trauma, with or without fracture • Trauma patients may have unknown baseline nerve injury • Impaired consciousness and distracting injury complicate assessment for preexisting nerve injury • Theoretic concern of "double-crush" phenomenon causing permanent injury if block performed on an already injured nerve • PNB possibly interferes with subsequent neurologic assessment by trauma/surgical team	• Perform and document careful neurologic assessment before performing any neuraxial or PNB • Avoid PNB at preexisting injury site • Consider alternate analgesic modes when nerve function is unknown • Coordinate with trauma and surgical team to clarify plans for further neurologic assessment; consider placing nerve catheter but not injecting local anesthetic until after neurological assessment is completed • Consider use of short-acting, low-dose local anesthetics to facilitate more rapid block regression if examination becomes necessary

Compartment syndrome	• Certain patterns and mechanisms of injury increase risk for ACS, especially involving shaft of tibia or radius • Diagnosis of ACS requires frequent, vigilant examination • Failure to diagnose ACS early can result in permanent injury, tissue loss, or amputation • Historic hesitation to offer PNB to patients with ACS risk due to concern of masking early symptoms	• Discuss individual patient risks for ACS with trauma/surgical team • Discuss alternate analgesic modes if PNB is not desired • If using continuous PNB, consider low-concentration, short-acting local anesthetic infusions • Ischemic pain usually still readily detected with low-density PNB • Recent evidence suggesting low-density PNB may actually aid in early ACS detection from ischemic breakthrough pain in an otherwise previously effective analgesic block
Infection risk	• Trauma patients are at increased risk of infection of any type • No large cohort analyses describe overall neuraxial or PNB infection risk factors in trauma patients • Injured extremities may have skin breakdown near desired block site, potentially increasing infection risk • Stress response to trauma (leukocytosis and low-grade fever) may mimic signs of systemic infection	• Assess for signs of local or systemic infection before block placement • Maintain sterile technique for all neuraxial or PNB procedures • Examine PNB catheter sites at regular intervals for early signs of infection • Consider catheter removal if patient's overall infection risk has greatly increased

Abbreviations: ACS, acute compartment syndrome; ATLS, advanced trauma life support; DVT, deep venous thrombosis; PNB, peripheral nerve block.

Table 3
Specific block techniques and considerations in acute trauma

Body Region	Block	Indications/Benefits	Special Considerations in Acute Trauma
Head and neck			
	Branches of trigeminal, deep/ superficial cervical plexus, occipital nerves	Irrigation and repair of lacerations to head, face, neck	• Horner syndrome may confuse examination of evolving brain injury • Need operator with detailed head/neck neuroanatomy expertise • Many injuries are amenable to field block by surgeon
Thorax			
Midline or bilateral chest	High thoracic epidural	• Reliable coverage of large anatomic areas • Visceral analgesia	• Sympathectomy may jeopardize safety in hypovolemic patient • Contraindicated in coagulopathy, hypovolemia, spine fracture, high ICP • Positioning limitations and access for block placement • Theoretic spinal cord blood flow compromise in spine trauma • Possible increased risk of deep vein thrombosis and length of stay
Unilateral chest injuries	Paravertebral	• Similar coverage to epidural, but with selective laterality and lower risk of sympathectomy or epidural hematoma	• Coagulopathy and risk of occult bleeding • Positioning limitations and access for block placement • Pneumothorax risk could further compromise respiratory function (less problematic in patients with preexisting chest tube) • Possible neuraxial spread could cause sympathectomy • Ultrasound may facilitate successful placement • Bilateral injuries can be addressed with bilateral blocks

Anatomic region	Block	Uses/Advantages	Considerations
Anterior chest wall, distal clavicle, axilla	• Serratus anterior plane (SA) • Pectoral plane (PEC I and PEC II) • Erector spinae plane (ES)	• Possible role for anterior rib fractures (SA), clavicle fractures (PEC), and chest tube pain (SA, ES) or posterior and lateral injuries (ES) • Anterior approach (for PEC, SA) is superficial and compressible • Ultrasound speeds learning techniques (SA, PEC, ES)	• Limited data in trauma population • Coverage may vary • Further study needed to describe roles of specific blocks for certain injury types
	Intercostal nerves	• Temporary analgesia for selected number of ribs • Chest tube placement	• For multiple rib fractures, multiple blocks may lead to LAST • Pneumothorax risk could further compromise respiratory function • Ultrasound may be useful diagnostic confirmatory tool to localize fracture and improve block accuracy • Increased local anesthetic absorption increases LAST risk and limits use of technique • Other techniques with lower LAST risk are likely preferable
	Intrapleural	• Selective laterality • Avoids sympathectomy	
Abdomen/pelvis/acetabulum			
Midline or bilateral lower trunk	Low thoracic epidural	• Reliable coverage of large anatomic areas • Visceral analgesia	• Contraindicated in coagulopathy, hypovolemia, spine fracture, high ICP • Position for block placement may not be feasible in acute trauma • Theoretic spinal cord blood flow compromise in spine trauma
Anterior abdominal wall	• Rectus abdominis sheath (RA) • Transversus abdominis plane (TAP) • Ilioinguinal/iliohypogastric	• May help post-laparotomy tidal volumes (RA, TAP) • Avoids neuraxial risks/side effects • Anterior approaches; superficial and compressible • Ultrasound speeds learning techniques	• Trauma or surgery may complicate tissue plane identification • Injuries, incisions, dressings, drains may impede access • Bilateral large-volume LA injection increases LAST risk • Visceral pain not covered • Coverage may vary • Limited data in trauma population

(continued on next page)

Table 3
(continued)

Body Region	Block	Indications/Benefits	Special Considerations in Acute Trauma
Low thoracic to hip	Quadratus lumborum	• Able to perform in supine position • Potential supra-umbilical and infra-umbilical coverage • Possible component of visceral coverage • Reported coverage of acetabulum and femoral neck	• Trauma or surgery may complicate tissue plane identification • Depth of target and proximity to retroperitoneum and kidneys poses risk of renal or colon puncture or retroperitoneal bleeding; consider other analgesic approaches in coagulopathic patients • Coverage may vary • Limited data in trauma population
Upper extremity			
Shoulder girdle and upper arm	Brachial plexus: interscalene approach	• Covers distal clavicle • Shoulder fracture or dislocation; can facilitate reduction • Humeral fractures	• Cervical immobilization impedes access to neck and limits head rotation for optimal block placement; ultrasound may help • Horner syndrome may confuse examination of evolving brain injury • Hemidiaphragm paralysis is likely; may exacerbate respiratory compromise, especially with contralateral thoracic trauma; consider targeted low-volume block or other approaches to brachial plexus • Dilute low-volume block may facilitate nerve function examination after reduction
Upper arm to digits	Brachial plexus: Supraclavicular approach	• Rapid analgesia for most of arm/hand • Immobilizes freshly repaired structures and provides regional sympathectomy after limb or digit salvage procedures	• Lower incidence of hemidiaphragm paralysis than interscalene, but consider same possible consequences • Easiest to perform with arm at side or adducted across body; can be quite challenging if pain precludes this positioning • Preexisting subcutaneous emphysema (as in some pneumothoraces) can interfere with ultrasound visualization • Inadvertent arterial puncture poses difficulty for hemostasis

Region	Technique	Advantages	Considerations
Elbow to digits	Brachial plexus: infraclavicular approach	• Usually spares phrenic nerve • Greater depth of target may improve nerve catheter fixation	• Inadvertent arterial puncture poses difficulty for hemostasis • Consider other approaches if in proximity to known vascular injury or central venous catheter insertion site
Forearm to digits	Brachial plexus: axillary approach	• Avoids phrenic nerve palsy • Can select nerves for targeted analgesia	• Placement requires arm abduction, possibly limited by pain • Transarterial approach risks impeding distal blood flow • Block site may be covered by dressing or splint
	Midhumeral and forearm blocks of radial, median, and ulnar nerves	• Can block specific nerves for selective analgesia • Preserves upper arm motor function	
Hand, digits	Intravenous regional (Bier block)	• Targeted hand/digit anesthesia for short procedures • Easy to learn, quick to perform • Preserves upper arm motor function	• Requires exsanguination of limb with Esmarch bandage; existing injuries can make this quite painful (may need brief sedation) • Tourniquet use required for block function; tourniquet pain may be intolerable and require sedation, higher risk if full stomach • Relies on short procedure duration; procedures outlasting block need LA supplementation, sedation, or GA conversion • Need alternate postoperative analgesia strategy, as block resolves at tourniquet deflation
Lower extremity			
Bilateral lower extremities and pelvis	Lumbar epidural	• Reliable coverage of large anatomic areas • Useful in bilateral lower extremity or pelvic trauma	• Contraindicated in coagulopathy, hypovolemia, spine fracture, high ICP • Position for block placement may not be feasible in acute trauma • Theoretic risk of compromised spinal cord blood flow with coexisting spine trauma
Acetabulum, proximal thigh, femur, knee	Lumbar plexus – psoas compartment	• Selective laterality • Covers entire lower extremity when combined with proximal sciatic block	• Position for block placement may not be feasible in acute trauma • Deep transmuscular approach is often painful; consider sedation risks if full stomach • Approach risks renal puncture, retroperitoneal bleed, or neuraxial spread; consider alternatives in coagulopathy or hypovolemia • Selective femoral, obturator, and lateral femoral cutaneous, or fascia iliaca block may be more appropriate when analgesia is desired distal to femoral head

(continued on next page)

Table 3
(continued)

Body Region	Block	Indications/Benefits	Special Considerations in Acute Trauma
Anterior and lateral thigh, hip, femur, knee, lower leg	• Fascia iliaca block (FIB) • Femoral nerve block (FNB) • Lateral femoral cutaneous nerve (LFCN) • Quadratus lumborum (QL)	• FIB: easy to learn, minimal equipment; option for prehospital or ED care • FNB: easy access in supine patient; fast • FIB/FNB/QL for hip fractures • FIB/FNB: excellent for mid- and distal femur, also for femoral/tibial traction pins; may need LFCN for lateral coverage	• Quadriceps motor block impairs ambulation; counsel patients about increased fall risk (FNB, FIB) • Consider adductor canal block for injury at or distal to knee • Use of dilute LA may offer analgesia with less motor block • Use of very dense LA could mask compartment syndrome of the thigh in high-risk injury patterns (FIB, FNB) • Limited data in acute trauma, but promising for further study in hip/acetabulum/proximal femur injury (QL)
Knee/Medial lower leg, ankle, foot	Adductor canal/subsartorial	• Pure sensory block • Preserves quadriceps function, allowing better mobility	• Target adjacent to large vessels and is deep, difficult to compress in coagulopathy • Consider more superficial block in coagulopathy (FNB or superficial saphenous approach distal to knee)
Posterior hip, thigh, femur, knee, lower leg, foot (except saphenous distribution)	Sciatic nerve (parasacral, transgluteal, infragluteal, anterior inguinal, midfemoral, popliteal)	• Multiple approach options depending on location of injury or surgery • Coverage distal to tibial plateau, offers complete lower extremity analgesia in combination with saphenous or FNB • Facilitates ankle reduction in ED • Anterior inguinal, infragluteal, midfemoral, and popliteal approach allow supine position	• Some approaches are deep, noncompressible, higher risk in coagulopathy • When target is deep, ultrasound imaging may be difficult; nerve stimulation possible but can increase pain in injured limb • Motor block of hamstring in proximal approaches limits crutch use; counsel patients about increased fall risk • Lateral or prone position needed for very proximal approaches; may not be feasible in acute trauma • Concern over use of very dense LA masking compartment syndrome of lower leg in high-risk injury patterns (tibial plateau/shaft fractures) • Frequent, meticulous compartment monitoring, in coordination with primary team, may permit dilute LA infusions for somatic analgesia while not blocking ischemic pain (controversy exists)
Midfoot, toes	Ankle block	• Major or minor procedures on foot • Ultrasound optional	• Need multiple injections for complete coverage; may be more unpleasant for patient • If tourniquet is needed, should consider more proximal block or added sedation

Abbreviations: ED, emergency department; GA, general anesthesia; ICP, intracranial pressure; LA, local anesthetic; LAST, local anesthetic systemic toxicity.

PNB in the anesthetized trauma patient is performed on a case-by-case basis in the authors' institutions.

PRIORITIZING RESUSCITATION

Measures to preserve life and avoid secondary injury take priority in the management of trauma patients. A systematic approach to initial patient assessment is well-defined and standardized through advanced trauma life support (ATLS) protocols and decision-making algorithms. Although regional block may be an elegant technique, it does take time and adequate resources (eg, personnel, equipment, and space) to safely perform. Not uncommonly, the degree of patients' emotional or physiologic distress may be so significant that induction of general anesthesia and airway securement are necessary to safely complete the primary and secondary surveys and initiate immediate resuscitative pathways in trauma.

POSITIONING LIMITATIONS

In general, block techniques that require a posterior approach may be difficult or impossible due to the need for supine positioning during most of the ATLS primary and secondary survey, and often for many hours after beginning initial resuscitation. Cervical immobilization may make interscalene and supraclavicular blocks more challenging with an inability to turn the neck to the contralateral side. Block approaches that require limb manipulation, such as the axillary approach to the brachial plexus, and subgluteal or popliteal approaches to the sciatic nerve, can be extremely painful in patients with extremity fractures. In many cases, ultrasound guidance may allow for rapid visualization of the targeted neural structures or an alternate approach with minimal or no need of modifying patient position. Finally, when modification of an injured patient's position is necessary for a regional technique, it is highly recommended to set up all the needed equipment in advance of patient positioning for efficiency and to minimize patient discomfort from unnecessarily prolonged block performance.

COAGULOPATHY

Although clinically significant bleeding events from regional block procedures are rare, they can occasionally produce devastating permanent injury when perineural bleeding occurs after neuraxial or deep intramuscular procedures, such as lumbar plexus block.[61] With many people taking newer anticoagulants and antiplatelet agents due to chronic medical conditions, acute trauma patients may have coagulopathies that are undetectable by routine blood and coagulation testing. Additionally, patients with severe injuries may have coagulopathy due to hemorrhage, hemodilution, hypothermia, brain injury, or acute coagulopathy of trauma.[62] Therefore, these deep blocks should be avoided in the presence or suspicion of coagulopathy, or when the prescription drug history of a patient cannot be determined. Some practitioners will consider placing non-neuraxial, superficial PNB in the presence of mild coagulopathy after appropriate discussion of risks and benefits with the patient or surrogate.[63] Case series data have reported safety of performing PNB in arthroplasty patients who then receive rivaroxaban prophylaxis, and for catheter removal in anticoagulated patients, although data from trauma populations are not available.[64] At present, there is insufficient evidence to quantify any alteration in bleeding risk when blocks are performed under ultrasound guidance versus blind approaches.

NERVE INJURY

Recognition of preexisting nerve injuries and avoiding secondary injury are important considerations in the acute trauma setting. A subset of trauma patients presents with acute nerve injury either via direct nerve involvement or secondary trauma to associ- ated structures, such as radial nerve palsies from humeral shaft fractures or peroneal nerve injuries after fibular fractures. Controversy exists as to whether proximal block of an injured nerve may lead to the "double-crush" phenomenon with increased risk of permanent neuropathy; however, clinical practice does not bear witness to these claims. It is vital that a sensory and motor assessment is conducted before performing a block, as some preexisting nerve deficits may not have been recognized yet by the patient or members of the team. Other injury patterns pose increased risk for intrao- perative iatrogenic injury. In some cases, with clear communication among all care providers, it may still be appropriate to perform PNB with a dilute, short-acting local anesthetic that allows for earlier block regression and functional assessment.

COMPARTMENT SYNDROME

High-energy or ballistic injuries with significant soft tissue damage or vascular injuries to the extremities, as well as some fracture patterns and operative repair may place trauma patients at increased risk of developing acute compartment syndrome (ACS). Tibial and radial fractures are among the most common orthopedic injuries, with ACS rates reportedly as high as 8.1% of patients with tibial diaphyseal fracture in 1 retrospective study.[65] Although conventional teaching has implicated regional an- esthetics in masking the initial symptoms of disproportionate pain and thus have discouraged nerve blocks in these patients, recent articles have countered by sug- gesting that dilute local anesthetic solutions via continuous PNB can in fact aid the early detection of ACS.[66] Ultimately, ACS remains a diagnosis of vigilance where frequent serial examinations are necessary for the timely detection and intervention of ACS in trauma patients. Collaborative decision-making and predetermined ACS protocols are vital to plan pain management strategies that allow for early compart- ment syndrome identification without resulting in undue patient suffering.

INFECTION RISK

Infections from single-injection or continuous PNB are uncommon events in non- trauma patients, with reported rates between 0% and 3%.[67-70] However, there is reason for heightened concern in trauma victims who may be prone to infection due to penetrating injuries, nonsterile emergent procedures, iatrogenic interventions, altered immune responses and perfusion, blood component transfusion, and mechan- ical ventilation. Findings of low-grade fever and leukocytosis are not unusual in trauma patients, and warrant appropriate laboratory investigation and physical examination when assessing PNB candidacy to evaluate an infectious etiology versus a normal physiologic trauma stress response. Furthermore, in the more critically ill trauma pa- tient who is at increased risk for nosocomial infection, it is important to conduct daily reappraisal of the risks and benefits provided by the PNB.

Infection data for regional anesthesia in trauma are sparse. Walter Reed Army Med- ical Center reported 7 (1.9%) of a cohort of 361 trauma patients with a continuous PNB developed a related infection, all being superficial skin infections that resolved with catheter removal.[71] In combat care, longer duration of an indwelling nerve catheter (4–11 days) was associated with risk of infection in a 5-case series of soldiers for whom nerve catheters were placed with sterile technique.[72] An assessment of bacterial cultures from the tips of epidural and peripheral nerve catheters from UK military personnel showed colonization in 34% and 29% of catheters, respectively, but only 1 patient with a positive catheter-tip culture had a clinically confirmed infection.[73] Recently, the American Society of Anesthesiologists and ASRA issued a joint practice advisory on infectious complications of neuraxial procedures, with recommendations about patient selection, skin preparation, aseptic technique, and postprocedure care of neuraxial catheters.[74] With insufficient evidence at present to guide specific practices to minimize infectious complications of PNB, trauma providers should be aware of this advisory and similarly incorporate vigilant sterile technique, serially examine the site of PNB catheters, and regularly assess for local and systemic infections in trauma patients.

FUTURE DIRECTIONS

Not all trauma care systems have staffing models to support extensive anesthesiology involvement in early resuscitation, outside of airway management and availability for emergent surgical needs. As trauma teams become more familiar with advantages of incorporating regional anesthetic techniques earlier in patient care, interest in developing expertise in these analgesic modalities is likely to grow, particularly in fields outside of anesthesiology.

Physician anesthesiologists are poised to lead other health professionals, not only in key principles of patient assessment for block candidacy and technical aspects of procedure performance, but in refining trauma pathways to include considerations of regional anesthetic options to improve patient comfort and potentially avoid problematic side effects of other interventions. With appropriate medical training, there may be a new role for teaching prehospital providers block techniques for select patterns of injury.

Additionally, more regional anesthesia experience in trauma should yield outcome data for circumstances when PNB has greatest benefit. In the present opioid epidemic, data about posttraumatic chronic pain and opioid use and dependence will clarify whether PNB can make an impact on this important public health issue.

SUMMARY

PNB can be challenging in trauma due to competing priorities in early resuscitation and surgical care, and due to the complexity of the polytrauma patient. In many instances, PNB offers a more favorable side-effect profile than systemic opioids and often provides superior analgesia. Because of these advantages, further research is warranted to assess the impact of PNB for specific indications in trauma, with attention to surgical outcomes, LOS, development of chronic pain, and opioid dependence. The rapid expansion of ultrasound availability in the past decade and increasing provider comfort with use of this technology for multiple point-of-care purposes have generated broader interest in learning ultrasound-guided nerve blocks. Prehospital and emergency medicine providers are important partners with anesthesiology-trained members of the trauma care team in bringing the advantages of regional anesthetic techniques to a greater proportion of trauma victims.

REFERENCES

1. Burke WC. Hydrochlorate of cocaine in minor surgery. NY Med J 1884;40:616–7.
2. Mulroy MF. Daniel C. Moore, MD, and the renaissance of regional anesthesia in North America. Reg Anesth Pain Med 2011;36(6):625–9.

3. Gelfand HJ, Kent ML, Buckenmaier CC 3rd. Management of acute pain of the war wounded during short and long-distance transport and "Casevac". Tech Orthop 2017;32(4):263–9.

4. Todd KH. A review of current and emerging approaches to pain management in the emergency department. Pain Ther 2017;6(2):193–202.

5. Gros T, Viel E, Ripart J, et al. Prehospital analgesia with femoral nerve block following lower extremity injury. A 107 cases survey. Ann Fr Anesth Reanim 2012;31(11):846–9 [in French].

6. Simpson PM, McCabe B, Bendall JC, et al. Paramedic-performed digital nerve block to facilitate field reduction of a dislocated finger. Prehosp Emerg Care 2012;16(3):415–7.

7. Dochez E, van Geffen GJ, Bruhn J, et al. Prehospital administered fascia iliaca compartment block by emergency medical service nurses, a feasibility study. Scand J Trauma Resusc Emerg Med 2014;22:38.

8. McRae PJ, Bendall JC, Madigan V, et al. Paramedic-performed fascia iliaca compartment block for femoral fractures: a controlled trial. J Emerg Med 2015; 48(5):581–9.

9. Wroe P, O'Shea R, Johnson B, et al. Ultrasound-guided forearm nerve blocks for hand blast injuries: case series and multidisciplinary protocol. Am J Emerg Med 2016;34(9):1895–7.

10. Clattenburg E, Herring A, Hahn C, et al. ED ultrasound-guided posterior tibial nerve blocks for calcaneal fracture analagesia. Am J Emerg Med 2016;34(6): 1183.e1-3.

11. Richman JM, Liu SS, Courpas G, et al. Does continuous peripheral nerve block provide superior pain control to opioids? A meta-analysis. Anesth Analg 2006; 102(1):248–57.

12. Blaivas M, Adhikari S, Lander L. A prospective comparison of procedural sedation and ultrasound-guided interscalene nerve block for shoulder reduction in the emergency department. Acad Emerg Med 2011;18(9):922–7.

13. Kent ML, Hsia HJ, Van de Ven TJ, et al. Perioperative pain management strategies for amputation: a topical review. Pain Med 2017;18(3):504–19.

14. Jenson MG, Sorensen RF. Early use of regional and local anesthesia in a combat environment may prevent the development of complex regional pain syndrome in wounded combatants. Mil Med 2006;171(5):396–8.

15. Taras JS, Behrman MJ. Continuous peripheral nerve block in replantation and revascularization. J Reconstr Microsurg 1998;14(1):17–21.

16. Liu Q, Chelly JE, Williams JP, et al. Impact of peripheral nerve block with low dose local anesthetics on analgesia and functional outcomes following total knee arthroplasty: a retrospective study. Pain Med 2015;16(5):998–1006.

17. Soberon JR Jr, Truxillo TM, Gethers CC, et al. Axillary block-induced chemical sympathectomy in the setting of digital ischemia. Ochsner J 2016;16(4):450–6.

18. Simon BJ, Cushman J, Barraco R, et al. Pain management guidelines for blunt thoracic trauma. J Trauma 2005;59(5):1256–67.

19. McKendy KM, Lee LF, Boulva K, et al. Epidural analgesia for traumatic rib fractures is associated with worse outcomes: a matched analysis. J Surg Res 2017;214:117–23.

20. Zaw AA, Murry J, Hoang D, et al. Epidural analgesia after rib fractures. Am Surg 2015;81(10):950–4.

21. Bossolasco M, Bernardi E, Fenoglio LM. Continuous serratus plane block in a patient with multiple rib fractures. J Clin Anesth 2017;38:85–6.

22. Kunhabdulla NP, Agarwal A, Gaur A, et al. Serratus anterior plane block for multiple rib fractures. Pain Physician 2014;17(4):E553–5.
23. Hamilton DL, Manickam B. Erector spinae plane block for pain relief in rib fractures. Br J Anaesth 2017;118(3):474–5.
24. Malekpour M, Hashmi A, Dove J, et al. Analgesic choice in management of rib fractures: paravertebral block or epidural analgesia? Anesth Analg 2017; 124(6):1906–11.
25. Mohta M, Verma P, Saxena AK, et al. Prospective, randomized comparison of continuous thoracic epidural and thoracic paravertebral infusion in patients with unilateral multiple fractured ribs–a pilot study. J Trauma 2009;66(4): 1096–101.
26. Truitt MS, Murry J, Amos J, et al. Continuous intercostal nerve blockade for rib fractures: ready for primetime? J Trauma 2011;71(6):1548–52 [discussion: 1552].
27. Galvagno SM Jr, Smith CE, Varon AJ, et al. Pain management for blunt thoracic trauma: a joint practice management guideline from the Eastern Association for the Surgery of Trauma and Trauma Anesthesiology Society. J Trauma Acute Care Surg 2016;81(5):936–51.
28. Carrier FM, Turgeon AF, Nicole PC, et al. Effect of epidural analgesia in patients with traumatic rib fractures: a systematic review and meta-analysis of randomized controlled trials. Can J Anaesth 2009;56(3):230–42.
29. Trelles Centurion M, Van Den Bergh R, Gray H. Anesthesia provision in disasters and armed conflicts. Curr Anesthesiol Rep 2017;7(1):1–7.
30. Gros T, Dareau S, Causse L, et al. Sciatic nerve block in prehospital care without nerve stimulator. Ann Fr Anesth Reanim 2007;26:381–3 [in French].
31. Gros T, Delire V, Dareau S, et al. Interscalene brachial plexus block in prehospital medicine. Ann Fr Anesth Reanim 2008;27:859–60.
32. Murata H, Salviz EA, Chen S, et al. Case report: ultrasound-guided continuous thoracic paravertebral block for outpatient acute pain management of multilevel unilateral rib fractures. Anesth Analg 2013;116(1):255–7.
33. Albrecht E, Taffe P, Yersin B, et al. Undertreatment of acute pain (oligoanalgesia) and medical practice variation in prehospital analgesia of adult trauma patients: a 10 yr retrospective study. Br J Anaesth 2013;110(1):96–106.
34. Kircher J, Drendel AL, Newton AS, et al. Pediatric musculoskeletal pain in the emergency department: a medical record review of practice variation. CJEM 2014;16(6):449–57.
35. Ritsema TS, Kelen GD, Pronovost PJ, et al. The national trend in quality of emergency department pain management for long bone fractures. Acad Emerg Med 2007;14(2):163–9.
36. Heilman JA, Tanski M, Burns B, et al. Decreasing time to pain relief for emergency department patients with extremity fractures. BMJ Qual Improv Rep 2016;5(1) [pii:u209522.w7251].
37. Agency for Healthcare Research and Quality. Emergency department (ED): median time from ED arrival to time of initial oral, intranasal or parenteral pain medication administration for ED patients with a principal diagnosis of long bone fracture. 2016. Available at: https://www.qualitymeasures.ahrq.gov/summaries/ summary/49600. Accessed January 15, 2018.
38. Joint Commission Resources. Comprehensive accreditation manual for hospitals. Oak Brook (IL): Joint Commission Resources; 2017.
39. Yaster M, Benzon HT, Anderson TA. "Houston, we have a problem!": the role of the anesthesiologist in the current opioid epidemic. Anesth Analg 2017;125(5): 1429–31.

40. Harford TC, Yi HY, Chen CM, et al. Substance use disorders and self- and other-directed violence among adults: results from the National Survey on Drug Use And Health. J Affect Disord 2018;225:365–73.

41. Cherpitel CJ, Ye Y, Andreuccetti G, et al. Risk of injury from alcohol, marijuana and other drug use among emergency department patients. Drug Alcohol Depend 2017;174:121–7.

42. Kumar K, Kirksey MA, Duong S, et al. A review of opioid-sparing modalities in perioperative pain management: methods to decrease opioid use postoperatively. Anesth Analg 2017;125(5):1749–60.

43. Beaudoin FL, Haran JP, Liebmann O. A comparison of ultrasound-guided three-in-one femoral nerve block versus parenteral opioids alone for analgesia in emergency department patients with hip fractures: a randomized controlled trial. Acad Emerg Med 2013;20(6):584–91.

44. Stewart B, Tudur Smith C, Teebay L, et al. Emergency department use of a continuous femoral nerve block for pain relief for fractured femur in children. Emerg Med J 2007;24(2):113–4.

45. Dickman E, Pushkar I, Likourezos A, et al. Ultrasound-guided nerve blocks for intracapsular and extracapsular hip fractures. Am J Emerg Med 2016;34(3):586–9.

46. Heflin T, Ahern T, Herring A. Ultrasound-guided infraclavicular brachial plexus block for emergency management of a posterior elbow dislocation. Am J Emerg Med 2015;33(9):1324.e1-4.

47. Tezel O, Kaldirim U, Bilgic S, et al. A comparison of suprascapular nerve block and procedural sedation analgesia in shoulder dislocation reduction. Am J Emerg Med 2014;32(6):549–52.

48. Stone MB, Wang R, Price DD. Ultrasound-guided supraclavicular brachial plexus nerve block vs procedural sedation for the treatment of upper extremity emergencies. Am J Emerg Med 2008;26(6):706–10.

49. O'Donnell BD, Ryan H, O'Sullivan O, et al. Ultrasound-guided axillary brachial plexus block with 20 milliliters local anesthetic mixture versus general anesthesia for upper limb trauma surgery: an observer-blinded, prospective, randomized, controlled trial. Anesth Analg 2009;109(1):279–83.

50. Gregoretti C, Decaroli D, Piacevoli Q, et al. Analgo-sedation of patients with burns outside the operating room. Drugs 2008;68(17):2427–43.

51. Diakomi M, Papaioannou M, Mela A, et al. Preoperative fascia iliaca compartment block for positioning patients with hip fractures for central nervous blockade: a randomized trial. Reg Anesth Pain Med 2014;39(5):394–8.

52. Sia S, Pelusio F, Barbagli R, et al. Analgesia before performing a spinal block in the sitting position in patients with femoral shaft fracture: a comparison between femoral nerve block and intravenous fentanyl. Anesth Analg 2004;99(4):1221–4 [Table of contents].

53. Schley M, Topfner S, Wiech K, et al. Continuous brachial plexus blockade in combination with the NMDA receptor antagonist memantine prevents phantom pain in acute traumatic upper limb amputees. Eur J Pain 2007;11(3):299–308.

54. Aitken E, Jackson A, Kearns R, et al. Effect of regional versus local anaesthesia on outcome after arteriovenous fistula creation: a randomised controlled trial. Lancet 2016;388(10049):1067–74.

55. Neal JM, Barrington MJ, Brull R, et al. The second ASRA practice advisory on neurologic complications associated with regional anesthesia and pain medicine: executive summary 2015. Reg Anesth Pain Med 2015;40:401–30. United States.

56. Kao MC, Tsai SK, Tsou MY, et al. Paraplegia after delayed detection of inadvertent spinal cord injury during thoracic epidural catheterization in an anesthetized elderly patient. Anesth Analg 2004;99(2):580–3 [Table of contents].

57. Benumof JL. Permanent loss of cervical spinal cord function associated with interscalene block performed under general anesthesia. Anesthesiology 2000; 93(6):1541–4.

58. Bromage PR, Benumof JL. Paraplegia following intracord injection during attempted epidural anesthesia under general anesthesia. Reg Anesth Pain Med 1998; 23(1):104–7.

59. Marhofer P. Regional blocks carried out during general anesthesia or deep sedation: myths and facts. Curr Opin Anaesthesiol 2017;30(5):621–6.

60. Taenzer AH, Walker BJ, Bosenberg AT, et al. Asleep versus awake: does it matter? Pediatric regional block complications by patient state: a report from the Pediatric Regional Anesthesia Network. Reg Anesth Pain Med 2014;39(4):279–83.

61. Weller RS, Gerancher JC, Crews JC, et al. Extensive retroperitoneal hematoma without neurologic deficit in two patients who underwent lumbar plexus block and were later anticoagulated. Anesthesiology 2003;98(2):581–5.

62. Chang R, Cardenas JC, Wade CE, et al. Advances in the understanding of trauma-induced coagulopathy. Blood 2016;128(8):1043–9.

63. Buckenmaier CC 3rd, Shields CH, Auton AA, et al. Continuous peripheral nerve block in combat casualties receiving low-molecular weight heparin. Br J Anaesth 2006;97(6):874–7.

64. Chelly JE, Metais B, Schilling D, et al. Combination of superficial and deep blocks with rivaroxaban. Pain Med 2015;16(10):2024–30.

65. Park S, Ahn J, Gee AO, et al. Compartment syndrome in tibial fractures. J Orthop Trauma 2009;23(7):514–8.

66. Nin OC, Patrick MR, Boezaart AP. The controversy of regional anesthesia, continuous peripheral nerve blocks, analgesia, and acute compartment syndrome. Tech Orthop 2017;32(4):243–7.

67. Horlocker TT, Abel MD, Messick JM Jr, et al. Small risk of serious neurologic complications related to lumbar epidural catheter placement in anesthetized patients. Anesth Analg 2003;96(6):1547–52 [Table of contents].

68. Bergman BD, Hebl JR, Kent J, et al. Neurologic complications of 405 consecutive continuous axillary catheters. Anesth Analg 2003;96(1):247–52 [Table of contents].

69. Cuvillon P, Ripart J, Lalourcey L, et al. The continuous femoral nerve block catheter for postoperative analgesia: bacterial colonization, infectious rate and adverse effects. Anesth Analg 2001;93(4):1045–9.

70. Capdevila X, Pirat P, Bringuier S, et al. Continuous peripheral nerve blocks in hospital wards after orthopedic surgery: a multicenter prospective analysis of the quality of postoperative analgesia and complications in 1,416 patients. Anesthesiology 2005;103(5):1035–45.

71. Stojadinovic A, Auton A, Peoples GE, et al. Responding to challenges in modern combat casualty care: innovative use of advanced regional anesthesia. Pain Med 2006;7(4):330–8.

72. Lai TT, Jaeger L, Jones BL, et al. Continuous peripheral nerve block catheter infections in combat-related injuries: a case report of five soldiers from Operation Enduring Freedom/Operation Iraqi Freedom. Pain Med 2011;12(11):1676–81.

73. Wood P, Gill M, Edwards D, et al. Clinical and microbiological evaluation of epidural and regional anaesthesia catheters in injured UK military personnel. J R Army Med Corps 2016;162(4):261–5.

74. Practice advisory for the prevention, diagnosis, and management of infectious complications associated with neuraxial techniques: an updated report by the American Society of Anesthesiologists Task Force on Infectious Complications Associated with Neuraxial Techniques and the American Society of Regional Anesthesia and Pain Medicine. Anesthesiology 2017;126(4):585–601.

Pediatric Ambulatory Continuous Peripheral Nerve Blocks

Sible Antony, MD[a], Harshad Gurnaney, MBBS, MPH[b],
Arjunan Ganesh, MBBS[b],*

KEYWORDS

- Pediatric regional anesthesia • Continuous peripheral nerve blockade • Ambulatory
- Peripheral nerve catheters • Complications

KEY POINTS

- Peripheral nerve blockade including continuous peripheral nerve blockade is gaining in popularity in pediatric anesthesia; however, ambulatory it is not commonly used in pediatric anesthesia practice.
- Surgical procedures that result in considerable pain beyond 24 hours may be indications for ambulatory continuous peripheral nerve blockade when appropriate.
- Use of ambulatory continuous peripheral nerve blockade in children has the potential to increase patient and family satisfaction and reduce postoperative costs and side effects.
- Although complications like pericatheter leakage, premature dislodgement, and block failure may occur, serious complication (permanent nerve injury, local anesthetic toxicity, infection) are rare.
- A dedicated program that includes selection of appropriate patients and procedures, aided by sound patient and family education and backed up by close regular follow-up is key to its success.

INTRODUCTION

Regional anesthetic techniques in children have been shown to help decrease postoperative opioid consumption and reduce side effects such as postoperative nausea and vomiting.[1] Single injection techniques, which are currently commonly used in most pediatric practices, only provide analgesia for 12 to 16 hours.[2] Although regional

Disclosure Statement: None.
[a] Department of Anesthesiology and Critical Care, The Children's Hospital of Philadelphia, 34th and Civic Center Boulevard, Philadelphia, PA 19104, USA; [b] Department of Anesthesiology and Critical Care, The Children's Hospital of Philadelphia, Perelman School of Medicine, University of Pennsylvania, 34th and Civic Center Boulevard, Philadelphia, PA 19104, USA
* Corresponding author.
E-mail address: Ganesha@email.chop.edu

Anesthesiology Clin 36 (2018) 455–465
https://doi.org/10.1016/j.anclin.2018.05.003
1932-2275/18/© 2018 Elsevier Inc. All rights reserved.

anesthesiology.theclinics.com

anesthesiologists can add analgesic adjuvants to help prolong the duration of this initial block, many operative procedures result in acute pain lasting beyond 16 hours. A potential solution to provide extended analgesia and decrease the length of stay in the hospital is through the use of continuous peripheral nerve blockade (CPNB). Although many pediatric practices have used CPNB for inpatient use, the use of ambulatory CPNB is very limited in pediatric practice.

Ambulatory CPNB have long been used for adult orthopedic procedures[3–5]; however, using home catheters for pediatric patients is still not very common.[6] Some of the challenges that may be encountered when using such catheters in pediatric patients are addressing concerns about safety in children, minimizing the risks of catheter dislodgement/leakage, patient/parent education, and maintaining appropriate follow-up while the catheter is in place or removed.

This review examines the current use of pediatric home catheters described in the literature. Common obstacles and complications encountered with existing home catheter techniques are also reviewed. As anesthesiologists in our current health care environment, we should be searching for ways to provide safe and cost-effective care for patients while improving patient satisfaction and expediting recovery.

INDICATIONS FOR OUTPATIENT PERIPHERAL NERVE CATHETERS

Ambulatory peripheral nerve catheters in the pediatric population are indicated for procedures where the pain from the operative procedure is expected to last longer than the duration of a single injection peripheral nerve block (about 12–20 hours).[7–11] Common strategies used to prolong the duration of a single injection block include increasing the concentration of the local anesthetic and use of additives (eg, clonidine, dexamethasone) to the local anesthetic injectate.[2,12,13] Even with these strategies, a single injection peripheral nerve block is unable to provide reliable analgesia beyond 20 hours. In these patients, CPNB provides an effective method to prolong the analgesic benefits of a peripheral nerve block for 48 to 72 hours postoperatively. Additional benefits from the use of CPNB include discharge home on the day of surgery, reduced postoperative opioid use, and improved patient satisfaction.[7,9,10,14]

Indications by Continuous Peripheral Nerve Blockade Location

Common indications for CPNB in pediatric patients include femoral CPNB for arthroscopic or open knee procedures, sciatic CPNB for foot and ankle procedures, lumbar plexus CPNB for major hip surgery, interscalene for shoulder rotator cuff repairs, and infraclavicular for major reconstruction in the upper extremity at or below the distal humerus[9,11,15,16] (Table 1). One of the areas of increasing interest has been the use of ambulatory thoracic paravertebral catheters for pectus excavatum repair surgery and other operative procedures.[17,18] There is a case series reporting the use of transversus abdominis plane block for lower abdominal procedures in pediatric patients in the inpatient setting.[19]

TECHNIQUES FOR PERIPHERAL NERVE CATHETERS
Ultrasound Guidance or Nerve Stimulation

The widespread use of ultrasound guidance to place the needle near the nerve, subsequently thread the perineural catheter, and confirm the location of the spread of the local anesthetic around the nerve has led to the question about the role of nerve stimulation in guiding the placement of a peripheral nerve catheter.[10,20–22] A recent meta-analysis reported a higher success rate of placement of the catheter and a lower risk of a vascular puncture when ultrasound guidance was compared with nerve stimulation.

Table 1
Indications for continuous peripheral nerve block catheters

Location of CPNB	Surgical Areas	Surgical Indications
Femoral	Knee and thigh	Knee (ligament reconstructions, tibial spine fracture, open meniscal repairs); femur osteotomy.
Adductor canal	Knee surgery	Arthroscopic knee procedures and for providing saphenous nerve analgesia to supplement a sciatic CPNB for below knee procedures.
Sciatic (popliteal)	Leg (below knee)	Calcaneal osteotomy/ORIF, midfoot osteotomy, placement of distal tibial and fibular external fixation device for leg lengthening procedures.
Lumbar plexus	Hip and thigh	Hip labrum repairs; femoral head and anterior thigh tumor resections.
Interscalene	Shoulder and proximal humerus	Shoulder arthroscopy with rotator cuff repair, Bankhart repair, and proximal humeral surgery.
Infraclavicular	Elbow, forearm, and hand	ORIF distal humerus, ORIF radius, ORIF ulna, arthroscopic or open elbow ligament repairs, major polydactyly repairs.
Paravertebral	Thoracic	Thoracotomy, Nuss procedure for pectus excavatum repair.

Abbreviations: CPNB, continuous peripheral nerve blockade; ORIF, open reduction and internal fixation.

However, no difference was reported in postoperative pain scores with movement.[22] A recent randomized, clinical trial with 450 patients randomized to either use of nerve stimulation for guiding the needle tip placement or stimulating catheter placement compared with ultrasound guidance only found that neither nerve stimulation groups was more effective in postoperative pain control than ultrasound guidance alone for femoral perineural catheter insertion.[23] Nevertheless, nerve stimulation can be used to supplement ultrasound guidance as a method to confirm needle to nerve proximity when the exact needle tip location may be difficult to discern, such as when performing deep blocks or when the person performing the CPNB is not as experienced with using ultrasound guidance for placement.

Ultrasound Guidance for Continuous Peripheral Nerve Blockade Placement (In-Plane Versus Out-of-Plane Technique)

When using ultrasound guidance to place a CPNB, the nerve can be visualized either in "long axis," with the length of the nerve positioned longitudinally within the ultrasound beam, or in "short axis," when viewed in cross-section. Also, the ultrasound probe orientation in relation to the needle can be either "in-plane," where the needle length is within a 2-dimensional ultrasound beam or "out-of-plane," where the needle length is through the ultrasound beam. For a majority of single-injection peripheral nerve blocks, the overwhelming majority of reports describe a short-axis view of the nerve with in-plane guidance of the needle. A potential disadvantage of this approach is that, when a catheter is threaded past the needle tip, it has a tendency in some locations to bypass the nerve, because the orientation of the catheter is now perpendicular to the nerve, depending on the catheter equipment used (eg, rigid catheter).[24–26] An advantage of this technique is that it is identical to the ultrasound-guided technique most commonly used for single-injection nerve blocks. Another approach is to guide the needle out of plane with the ultrasound field of view and the nerve visualized in the short axis. A potential disadvantage of this approach is that the needle tip is not always visualized, but the trajectory of the needle and eventual catheter deployment is nearly parallel to the target nerve, which allows a greater length of the catheter to remain in close proximity to the nerve as it is threaded past the needle tip.[27,28] In our experience, this approach allows for catheter placement in proximity to the nerve and allows 3 to 5 cm of the catheter to be threaded close to the nerve, which decreases the risk of dislodgement.[8,9] The choice of insertion technique should be made based on the equipment available as well as training and experience of the regional anesthesiologist.

Leakage Around the Continuous Peripheral Nerve Blockade Insertion Site

One of the concerns with the postoperative management of CPNB has been the concern about leakage of local anesthetic around the insertion site. This leads to soiling of the dressing and can lead to catheter dislodgment, the most common complication related to CPNB.[9,10,29] One strategy to decrease leakage around the catheter insertion site is to use 2-octyl cyanoacrylate glue (Dermabond Topical Skin Adhesive, Ethicon, Somerville, NJ) to secure the site of the CPNB catheter.[30] Another suggested technique has been to use a catheter-over-needle system, which places the perineural catheter over an insertion needle to decrease the incidence of leakage around the catheter insertion site.[31] However, this type of catheter equipment may have other disadvantages, depending on the insertion technique used.[32]

LOCAL ANESTHETIC INFUSIONS AND DELIVERY DEVICES
Type of Local Anesthetic

In pediatric regional anesthesiology, the most common local anesthetics used in perineural infusions are bupivacaine and ropivacaine, with a growing trend toward the latter recently.[9,10,33] Infusion rates and concentrations are based on the weight of the child, the location of the block, and the desired density of the block.[8,9] Studies performed in adults show that the primary determinant of efficacy and the extent of the motor blockade in lower extremity blocks is related to the total dose of local anesthetic and not solely based on the rate or concentration of infusate.[34–36] This has led to the suggestion that, if a longer duration of perineural infusions is desired, a combination of a higher concentration and lower rate may be used for lower extremity perineural infusions.[6] However, a similar effect has not been observed with upper extremity blocks.[6] The typical local anesthetics and concentrations used in pediatric practice are ropivacaine 0.10% to 0.2% and bupivacaine 0.10% to 0.25%.[7–10] Infusion rates may be determined by the location of the block, the position of the catheter relative to the target nerve or plexus, and the extent of block desired. In a study where ambulatory CPNB was used in various anatomic sites, the rate of ropivacaine used for pediatric CPNB ranged from 0.12 to 0.33 mg/kg/h.[10]

One of the most common indications for ambulatory pediatric perineural infusions is anterior cruciate ligament reconstruction, where a single injection sciatic block is performed along with continuous femoral perineural infusion.[7–10] A recent study evaluated the serum bupivacaine levels in children having this combination of blocks, where 0.25% bupivacaine was used for the bolus injections and the 0.10% bupivacaine (for 48 hours) was used for the infusions and did not observe toxic levels in any patient.[37] Although several adjuvants like opioids, clonidine, dexmedetomidine, midazolam, epinephrine, tramadol, and magnesium have been added to local anesthetics to prolong the duration of single injection blocks, they are unable to reliably extend analgesia beyond 24 hours. Therefore, if a longer duration of titratable regional anesthesia is desired, continuous perineural infusions should be used.[4]

Elastomeric and Electronic Infusion Pumps

Although elastomeric pumps are the most common pumps that have been used in ambulatory continuous perineural infusions,[7–10] the use of electronic pumps has been reported.[8,9] Electronic pumps are more versatile regarding the various delivery features and are also more accurate.[38] However, elastomeric pumps are easy to use, cheaper, and quieter.[38–40] Elastomeric pumps tend to deliver a higher rate, both at the start and toward the end of the infusion.[38] One needs to keep this in mind, particularly, in small children and when multiple perineural infusions are used for a single patient.[41] In a study comparing 2 elastomeric pumps, the Ambu Smart-Infuser Pain Pump (Ambu Inc., Columbia, MD) and the On-Q Pump with Select-a-Flow Variable Rate (I-Flow Corporation, Lake Forest, CA), it was observed that the On-Q pump (in the settings of normal fill and 150% overfill) delivered a significantly higher output per hour than the set rate during the first 8 hours, whereas the Ambu pump delivered a value closer to the set rate of 10 mL/h.[42]

POSTOPERATIVE MANAGEMENT
Instructions for the Family

Typically, the perineural infusions are started in the postanesthesia care unit.[10,33,41] All patients (and their family members) receive verbal and written instructions (**Fig. 1**) about safely removing the catheter and the recognition of potential complications before being discharged home.[8,9] The infusion pump manufacturer's information booklet is also provided for the family to take home. Patients and families are cautioned to avoid weight bearing on the extremities that could be weak (motor block) and to protect areas with a sensory block from injury (eg, from heat, cold, pressure, and other trauma). Instructions include clamping the catheter to pause the infusion in the case of an insensate extremity, local anesthetic toxicity, or excessive leakage.

At-Home Follow-Up

Typically, the patient's family member(s) remove peripheral nerve catheters at home. Contact information to reach the pain service is provided, and the family member(s) are instructed and encouraged to call the service if any questions arise regarding the CPNBs or postoperative pain control. All patients with CPNBs receive follow-up calls, usually by a member of the pain management service, to assess the effectiveness of pain management and answer any questions the family members may have regarding the CPNBs. Patients are prescribed adjuvant oral analgesics by the primary team[8,10] before discharge home. They are also asked to contact the pain service provider on call if they have any concerns with the CPNB or questions regarding the patient's pain management.[8,10]

SAFETY AND COMPLICATIONS

The safety profile of peripheral nerve catheters has been studied using the Pediatric Regional Anesthesia Network database. Although these results may not be extrapolated to children less than 3 years old, severe complications were rare with peripheral

The Children's Hospital *of* Philadelphia®
Hope lives here.®

28:B:15

Caring for Your Child
Peripheral Nerve Catheter Pain Control Device

Contact Number: If you have any questions or problems related to the pain control pump, or if your child's pain is not controlled, call 215-590-1000, and ask the operator to contact the pain management provider on call.

Call your surgeon/primary physician with any other questions about your child's care.

Many children go home with peripheral nerve catheters. **An adult trained in the care and use of the pump must be in the house during the nerve catheter infusion.** It is important to read the info below to know when to get help for your child.

In the unlikely event that your child has a seizure, close the clamp and call 911.

Close the clamp on the pump tubing to stop the infusion, and go to the nearest Emergency Room, if your child has any of the following symptoms:

- Numbness or tingling around the mouth
- Funny taste in the mouth
- Ringing, buzzing in ears
- Trembling
- General feeling that things are not right
- Increased irritability/inconsolable
- Blurred vision
- Confusion

Close the clamp on the pump tubing to stop the infusion and contact the pain management provider for any of the following:

- Redness, swelling, pain, or discharge at the nerve catheter site
- Excessive bleeding or drainage from the nerve catheter site.
- The catheter comes out or is disconnected (Do not attempt to push catheter in, or reconnect.)
- The arm/leg with the pain catheter is cool, blue, or swollen
- Unable to move the arm/leg with the pain catheter in it
- Numbness, tingling, extending beyond the arm or leg with the nerve catheter
- Dizziness, lightheadedness
- Nausea/vomiting

Fig. 1. Patient discharge instructions. (Images provided *courtesy of* Children's Hospital of Philadelphia. ©2018 The Children's Hospital of Philadelphia. Visit www.chop.edu for more information.)

nerve catheters and no local anesthetic toxicity was observed. The Pediatric Regional Anesthesia Network did report a 0.9% incidence of vascular punctures and a 0.6% incidence of excessive motor blockade as determined by the anesthesiologist. None of these complications had permanent sequelae. Catheters in place for more than 3 days had a higher incidence of insertion site infection.[29] An important distinction that the Pediatric Regional Anesthesia Network database failed to make is differentiating between inpatient and outpatient peripheral nerve catheters. A study from Gurnaney and colleagues,[9] based on nerve catheters in 1285 ambulatory pediatric patients, showed that 1283 patients were able to remain comfortable at home with oral opioids. There was no permanent neurologic injury detected. There was 1 instance of contralateral numbness after an interscalene catheter had been infusing for 17 hours. This numbness resolved within a few hours after the infusion was clamped. Although ultrasound guidance was used for this block, radiographic evidence of catheter tip

28:B:15

If your child has an upper extremity nerve catheter, and has loss of voice or difficulty swallowing, **close the clamp** on the pump tubing to stop the infusion and contact the pain management provider.

Special Instructions:
The peripheral nerve catheter causes your child's arm/leg to become numb or have decreased sensation. Your child can be injured if you don't protect the numb arm/leg. Talk with your doctor or nurse about how to protect the "numb" arm/leg from a pressure injury. Your child's arm (and fingers) or legs (and toes) should be able to move. Fingernails and toenails should be pink and warm.

- Avoid placing or spilling anything that is very hot or cold on or near the arm/leg with the pain catheter.
- Protect the affected area from pressure and sharp objects.
- No driving, bike riding, or use of heavy machinery.

Keep the pain pump close to your child at all times. This will help prevent pulling the nerve catheter out accidentally.

Dressings:
- Keep the nerve catheter dressing dry and intact.
- You will receive separate instructions for the surgical dressing.

Bath/Shower: Your child should not bathe/shower while the nerve catheter is in place. After it is removed, please follow the recommendation of your surgeon/physician.

Catheter Removal: There may be some medicine left in the pump when it is time to remove it.

1) Remove the clear nerve catheter dressing.
2) Gently pull out the tubing along the body toward the feet for leg surgery, (or toward the upper arm for arm/shoulder surgery.) Do not pull straight up (see picture to the right).
3) You will need to pull out about 3 inches of tubing, until you reach the end of the catheter. There is a gold or black tip on the end of the catheter.
4) A Band-Aid is usually not needed.

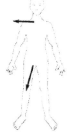

Written 11/16

Fig. 1. (continued).

location for this block was not available at the time of complaint to determine the exact etiology. Institutions across the country have various methods/standards for placement of these catheters as well as for outpatient follow-up. This variation may lead to the underreporting of certain complications such as paresthesia, numbness, or weakness.

In several single-center and multicenter studies conducted in children,[7–10,33,43] no permanent instances of nerve injury were noted. Complications during catheter placement such as inadvertent vascular injury, accidental placement, or migration into the epidural or intrathecal space are rare but possible. The most common complications that were reported include pericatheter leakage, premature dislodgement of the catheter, and inadequate analgesia.[8–10,33] There have been a few reported cases of possible local anesthetic toxicity where patients reported a metallic taste and ringing in their ears that resolved uneventfully after clamping and removal of the catheter.[8,9,33] Neurologic symptoms included paresthesia and patchy areas of numbness that resolved spontaneously within a few days to months.[9,43] Although falls related to femoral perineural infusions were reported in one of the pediatric studies,[10] the risk of falls is very rare in pediatric patients because most procedures in children that have continuous femoral perineural infusions are usually not allowed to fully weight bear.

CONTROVERSIES

There remains a difference of opinion between surgeons and anesthesiologists over the role of regional anesthesia in children at risk for acute compartment syndrome (ACS) after surgery. There is no evidence that CPNB in children masks ACS. Case reports and case series in children and adults have demonstrated that regional anesthesia does not contribute to a delay in or masking of the diagnosis of ACS.[11,44–46] A delay in the diagnosis of ACS is mostly caused by not properly identifying patients at risk along with insufficient postoperative monitoring of these patients.[47] It is suggested that, when considering CPNB in children at risk for ACS, lower concentrations of local anesthetics at lower rates be used (particularly for sciatic perineural catheters), with avoidance or cautious use of local anesthetic additives that may increase the density of the block.[47]

Performing regional anesthesia, particularly interscalene blocks in children under general anesthesia, was controversial in the past and was largely based on case reports.[48] However, based on data obtained from several case series, there is now a general agreement that performing pediatric regional anesthesia under general anesthesia/deep sedation is associated with acceptable safety and should be viewed as the standard of care.[15,43,47,49] Serious complications may still occur, even in experienced hands, and unexpected clinical outcomes must be aggressively investigated and managed.[47]

SUMMARY

CPNB in children for postoperative analgesia is gaining in popularity after several reports of efficacy and safety. Judicious patient and block selection followed by detailed patient and family education along with thorough follow-up will ensure the success of an ambulatory perineural catheter program. Advances in techniques and equipment and the ability for remote monitoring may further enhance safety and widespread use.

REFERENCES

1. Rose JB, Watcha MF. Postoperative nausea and vomiting in paediatric patients. Br J Anaesth 1999;83(1):104–17.
2. Cucchiaro G, Ganesh A. The effects of clonidine on postoperative analgesia after peripheral nerve blockade in children. Anesth Analg 2007;104(3):532–7.
3. Ilfeld BM. Continuous peripheral nerve blocks in the hospital and at home. Anesthesiol Clin 2011;29(2):193–211.
4. Ilfeld BM. Continuous peripheral nerve blocks: an update of the published evidence and comparison with novel, alternative analgesic modalities. Anesth Analg 2017;124(1):308–35.

5. Klein SM, Buckenmaier CC 3rd. Ambulatory surgery with long acting regional anesthesia. Minerva Anestesiol 2002;68(11):833–41, 841-837.
6. Machi AT, Ilfeld BM. Continuous peripheral nerve blocks in the ambulatory setting: an update of the published evidence. Curr Opin Anaesthesiol 2015; 28(6):648–55.
7. Dadure C, Bringuier S, Raux O, et al. Continuous peripheral nerve blocks for postoperative analgesia in children: feasibility and side effects in a cohort study of 339 catheters. Can J Anaesth 2009;56(11):843–50.
8. Ganesh A, Rose JB, Wells L, et al. Continuous peripheral nerve blockade for inpatient and outpatient postoperative analgesia in children. Anesth Analg 2007;105(5):1234–42 [table of contents].
9. Gurnaney H, Kraemer FW, Maxwell L, et al. Ambulatory continuous peripheral nerve blocks in children and adolescents: a longitudinal 8-year single center study. Anesth Analg 2014;118(3):621–7.
10. Visoiu M, Joy LN, Grudziak JS, et al. The effectiveness of ambulatory continuous peripheral nerve blocks for postoperative pain management in children and adolescents. Paediatr Anaesth 2014;24(11):1141–8.
11. Walker BJ, Noonan KJ, Bosenberg AT. Evolving compartment syndrome not masked by a continuous peripheral nerve block: evidence-based case management. Reg Anesth Pain Med 2012;37(4):393–7.
12. Chong MA, Berbenetz NM, Lin C, et al. Perineural versus intravenous dexamethasone as an adjuvant for peripheral nerve blocks: a systematic review and meta-analysis. Reg Anesth Pain Med 2017;42(3):319–26.
13. Jaeger P, Grevstad U, Koscielniak-Nielsen ZJ, et al. Does dexamethasone have a perineural mechanism of action? A paired, blinded, randomized, controlled study in healthy volunteers. Br J Anaesth 2016;117(5):635–41.
14. Dadure C, Motais F, Ricard C, et al. Continuous peripheral nerve blocks at home for treatment of recurrent complex regional pain syndrome I in children. Anesthesiology 2005;102(2):387–91.
15. Gurnaney H, Muhly WT, Kraemer FW, et al. Safety of pediatric continuous interscalene block catheters placed under general anesthesia: a single center's experience. Acta Anaesthesiol Scand 2015;59(3):377–83.
16. Hall-Burton DM, Hudson ME, Grudziak JS, et al. Regional anesthesia is cost-effective in preventing unanticipated hospital admission in pediatric patients having anterior cruciate ligament reconstruction. Reg Anesth Pain Med 2016;41(4): 527–31.
17. Vecchione T, Zurakowski D, Boretsky K. Thoracic paravertebral nerve blocks in pediatric patients: safety and clinical experience. Anesth Analg 2016;123(6): 1588–90.
18. Visoiu M. Outpatient analgesia via paravertebral peripheral nerve block catheter and On-Q pump–a case series. Paediatr Anaesth 2014;24(8):875–8.
19. Visoiu M, Boretsky KR, Goyal G, et al. Postoperative analgesia via transversus abdominis plane (TAP) catheter for small weight children-our initial experience. Paediatr Anaesth 2012;22(3):281–4.
20. Ponde VC, Desai AP, Shah DM, et al. Feasibility and efficacy of placement of continuous sciatic perineural catheters solely under ultrasound guidance in children: a descriptive study. Paediatr Anaesth 2011;21(4):406–10.
21. Bendtsen TF, Nielsen TD, Rohde CV, et al. Ultrasound guidance improves a continuous popliteal sciatic nerve block when compared with nerve stimulation. Reg Anesth Pain Med 2011;36(2):181–4.

22. Schnabel A, Meyer-Friessem CH, Zahn PK, et al. Ultrasound compared with nerve stimulation guidance for peripheral nerve catheter placement: a meta-analysis of randomized controlled trials. Br J Anaesth 2013;111(4):564–72.

23. Farag E, Atim A, Ghosh R, et al. Comparison of three techniques for ultrasound-guided femoral nerve catheter insertion: a randomized, blinded trial. Anesthesiology 2014;121(2):239–48.

24. Schwenk ES, Gandhi K, Baratta JL, et al. Ultrasound-guided out-of-plane vs. in-plane interscalene catheters: a randomized, prospective study. Anesth Pain Med 2015;5(6):e31111.

25. Ilfeld BM, Fredrickson MJ, Mariano ER. Ultrasound-guided perineural catheter insertion: three approaches but few illuminating data. Reg Anesth Pain Med 2010;35(2):123–6.

26. Ilfeld BM, Sandhu NS, Loland VJ, et al. Ultrasound-guided (needle-in-plane) perineural catheter insertion: the effect of catheter-insertion distance on postoperative analgesia. Reg Anesth Pain Med 2011;36(3):261–5.

27. Wang AZ, Gu L, Zhou QH, et al. Ultrasound-guided continuous femoral nerve block for analgesia after total knee arthroplasty: catheter perpendicular to the nerve versus catheter parallel to the nerve. Reg Anesth Pain Med 2010;35(2):127–31.

28. Mariano ER, Kim TE, Funck N, et al. A randomized comparison of long-and short-axis imaging for in-plane ultrasound-guided femoral perineural catheter insertion. J Ultrasound Med 2013;32(1):149–56.

29. Walker BJ, Long JB, De Oliveira GS, et al. Peripheral nerve catheters in children: an analysis of safety and practice patterns from the Pediatric Regional Anesthesia Network (PRAN). Br J Anaesth 2015;115(3):457–62.

30. Gurnaney H, Kraemer FW, Ganesh A. Dermabond decreases pericatheter local anesthetic leakage after continuous perineural infusions. Anesth Analg 2011;113(1):206.

31. Tsui BC, Ip VH. Catheter-over-needle method reduces risk of perineural catheter dislocation. Br J Anaesth 2014;112(4):759–60.

32. Steffel L, Howard SK, Borg L, et al. Randomized comparison of popliteal-sciatic perineural catheter tip migration and dislocation in a cadaver model using two catheter designs. Korean J Anesthesiol 2017;70(1):72–6.

33. Gable A, Burrier C, Stevens J, et al. Home peripheral nerve catheters: the first 24 months of experience at a children's hospital. J Pain Res 2016;9:1067–72.

34. Bauer M, Wang L, Onibonoje OK, et al. Continuous femoral nerve blocks: decreasing local anesthetic concentration to minimize quadriceps femoris weakness. Anesthesiology 2012;116(3):665–72.

35. Ilfeld BM, Moeller LK, Mariano ER, et al. Continuous peripheral nerve blocks: is local anesthetic dose the only factor, or do concentration and volume influence infusion effects as well? Anesthesiology 2010;112(2):347–54.

36. Madison SJ, Monahan AM, Agarwal RR, et al. A randomized, triple-masked, active-controlled investigation of the relative effects of dose, concentration, and infusion rate for continuous popliteal-sciatic nerve blocks in volunteers. Br J Anaesth 2015;114(1):121–9.

37. Suresh S, De Oliveira GS Jr. Blood bupivacaine concentrations after a combined single-shot sciatic block and a continuous femoral nerve block in pediatric patients: a prospective observational study. Anesth Analg 2017;124(5):1591–3.

38. Ilfeld BM, Morey TE, Enneking FK. The delivery rate accuracy of portable infusion pumps used for continuous regional analgesia. Anesth Analg 2002;95(5):1331–6 [table of contents].

39. Ilfeld BM, Morey TE, Enneking FK. Portable infusion pumps used for continuous regional analgesia: delivery rate accuracy and consistency. Reg Anesth Pain Med 2003;28(5):424–32.
40. Ilfeld BM, Morey TE, Enneking FK. Delivery rate accuracy of portable, bolus-capable infusion pumps used for patient-controlled continuous regional analgesia. Reg Anesth Pain Med 2003;28(1):17–23.
41. Ganesh A, Cucchiaro G. Multiple simultaneous perineural infusions for postoperative analgesia in adolescents in an outpatient setting. Br J Anaesth 2007;98(5): 687–9.
42. Iliev P, Bhalla T, Tobias JD. A comparison of the hourly output between the Ambu(R) smart-infuser pain pump and the On-Q Pump(R) with select-a-flow variable rate controller with standard and overfill volumes. Paediatr Anaesth 2016;26(4): 425–8.
43. Polaner DM, Taenzer AH, Walker BJ, et al. Pediatric Regional Anesthesia Network (PRAN): a multi-institutional study of the use and incidence of complications of pediatric regional anesthesia. Anesth Analg 2012;115(6):1353–64.
44. Dalens B. Some current controversies in paediatric regional anaesthesia. Curr Opin Anaesthesiol 2006;19(3):301–8.
45. Klucka J, Stourac P, Stouracova A, et al. Compartment syndrome and regional anaesthesia: critical review. Biomed Pap Med Fac Univ Palacky Olomouc Czech Repub 2017;161(3):242–51.
46. Kucera TJ, Boezaart AP. Regional anesthesia does not consistently block ischemic pain: two further cases and a review of the literature. Pain Med 2014; 15(2):316–9.
47. Lonnqvist PA, Ecoffey C, Bosenberg A, et al. The European society of regional anesthesia and pain therapy and the American society of regional anesthesia and pain medicine joint committee practice advisory on controversial topics in pediatric regional anesthesia I and II: what do they tell us? Curr Opin Anaesthesiol 2017;30(5):613–20.
48. Benumof JL. Permanent loss of cervical spinal cord function associated with interscalene block performed under general anesthesia. Anesthesiology 2000; 93(6):1541–4.
49. Taenzer A, Walker BJ, Bosenberg AT, et al. Interscalene brachial plexus blocks under general anesthesia in children: is this safe practice?: A report from the Pediatric Regional Anesthesia Network (PRAN). Reg Anesth Pain Med 2014;39(6): 502–5.

What Can Regional Anesthesiology and Acute Pain Medicine Learn from "Big Data"?

Nabil M. Elkassabany, MD, MSCE[a],*, Stavros G. Memtsoudis, MD, PhD[b],
Edward R. Mariano, MD, MAS (Clinical Research)[c]

KEYWORDS

• Big data • Outcomes • Regional anesthesia • Mortality • Anesthesia technique

KEY POINTS

• The concept of value-based health care is now reality for anesthesiology and surgery practices. Physicians practicing regional anesthesiology and acute pain medicine must demonstrate the value they add to patients' perioperative experience.

• Database research can provide good insight into rare outcomes and demonstrate effectiveness of regional anesthesiology and acute pain medicine interventions across different practice settings.

• This type of research may provide an alternative to the resource-intensive randomized clinical trials in certain situations and help generate hypotheses that can be further tested in prospective studies.

• Results of different types of research (prospective or retrospective) should be interpreted in the context of methodological limitations.

• Outcomes associated with regional anesthesiology and acute pain medicine that have been studied using "big data" include but are not limited to mortality and morbidity, resource utilization, surgical site infection, inpatient falls, and local anesthetic systemic toxicity.

• Results of these studies may inform health policy and decision making in terms of payment models and adoption of best practices.

[a] Sections of Orthopedic and Regional Anesthesiology, Department of Anesthesiology and Critical Care, University of Pennsylvania, 3400 Spruce Street, Dulles 6, Philadelphia, PA 19104, USA; [b] Department of Anesthesiology, Weill Cornell Medical College, Hospital for Special Surgery, 535 East 70th street, New York, NY 10021, USA; [c] Anesthesiology and Perioperative Care Service, VA Palo Alto Health Care System, Stanford University School of Medicine, 3801 Miranda Avenue, Palo Alto, CA 94304, USA
* Corresponding author.
E-mail address: Nabil.Elkassabany@uphs.upenn.edu

Anesthesiology Clin 36 (2018) 467–478
https://doi.org/10.1016/j.anclin.2018.04.003
1932-2275/18/© 2018 Elsevier Inc. All rights reserved.
anesthesiology.theclinics.com

INTRODUCTION

Value-based health care represents a delivery model in which providers, including hospitals and physicians, are paid based on the quality of care and costs of providing it rather than the volume of interventions. In the perioperative realm, providers are rewarded for helping patients improve their surgical outcomes, reduce postoperative complications, and decrease readmissions after surgery. Capturing outcome data about the results of each intervention has become a priority in this health care environment. In its effort to adapt to this new value-based model of health care delivery, the American Society of Anesthesiologists has promoted the Perioperative Surgical Home model in which physician anesthesiologists function as leaders in the coordination of perioperative care for surgical patients with the goal of improving outcomes.[1,2] Critics argue that anesthesiologists are not ready to take on this expanded role and question whether the financial aspects of this model are sustainable.[3-5] Alternative perioperative care models have been proposed, such as service line models,[6] where anesthesiologists play an integral role within an evidence-based care pathway but are not necessarily the sole leaders. Multiple enhanced recovery after surgery protocols have thrived within the latter model.[7] Irrespective of the care model and its name, it is clear that the unifying challenge continues to be the selection of outcomes and demonstration of improved quality attributable to the anesthesiologist's role and/or his/her choice of anesthetic or analgesic technique. In this context, it has traditionally been challenging to derive conclusive information from clinical studies due to the often rare nature of outcomes in question. The advent and evolution of large database research, however, facilitated by ever-increasing computing power and advances in methodology has allowed for analysis of large data constructs collected by an increasing number of hospitals, thus providing answers to important questions that previously seemed elusive. Therefore, this review addresses anesthesiologist-driven factors related to regional anesthesiology and acute pain medicine with an emphasis on selecting perioperative outcomes using big data and potential future directions that may influence research, clinical practice, and health policy.

PROS AND CONS OF BIG DATA RESEARCH

The major advantage of randomized clinical trials is that randomization and blinding provide reasonable protection against bias and confounding. Strict inclusion and exclusion criteria, however, are built into the structure of these trials, which may keep some patients who may benefit from the intervention from being enrolled. Consequently, patients who frequently represent problem cases in real-world practice are often not included, thus leaving results subject to questions of applicability in these populations. The fact that such studies are usually performed at academic institutions may limit external validity. Additionally, management pathways within the clinical trials are often detailed and enforced by the study protocol. These factors may limit the generalizability of the results to different patient populations or practice settings and even routine clinical practice at the same institution. Large randomized trials are expensive, resource intensive and time intensive, and sometimes marginally powered.

Studies of clinical and administrative databases use epidemiologic and statistical techniques to evaluate the effects of treatments in real-world situations. A major advantage of this approach is that the results come from data collected in routine clinical practice and may thus be more generalizable. Another advantage is that it allows study of rare outcomes/events and their association with perioperative patient-specific or surgery-specific variables. Database research suffers, however, from some inherent biases. Selection bias occurs when treatments are nonrandomly assigned, which is a normal part of clinical practice. Researchers are able to adjust for known patient and surgical factors through statistical models. The difficulty is that unknown or unexpected differences may contribute to an apparent effect of a given intervention. Measurement bias occurs when outcome assessments are either erroneous or miscoded or missing. Most of the databases are built for administrative or quality-improvement purposes and not for medical research. Researchers often capture outcomes through billing claims using diagnostic codes that may be subject to error or under-reporting. Confounding is another consideration in database research. It occurs when an intervention and an outcome are linked by a third factor. The downside is that the linking factor may not have been captured, or accounted for, in the database or may not even be known.

RARE OUTCOMES AND SOURCES OF BIG DATA

For anesthesiologists, avoiding adverse events of the lowest frequency (eg, death, recall, and nerve injury) tends to receive highest priority in the perioperative period, with fatal outcomes ranking first among complications to avoid.[8] This is not surprising, given that anesthesiology was the only medical specialty identified as making positive changes in terms of patient safety in the Institute of Medicine report, "To Err is Human: Building a Safer Health System."[9] Studies involving rare outcomes, positive or negative, invariably require accumulation of big data. Such studies must either involve multiple institutions over a long period (if prospective) or access data involving a large cohort of patients for retrospective analyses. These study designs involving longitudinal data may also require advanced statistical methods.[10] For example, Memtsoudis and colleagues[11] sought to evaluate postoperative morbidity and mortality for lower extremity joint arthroplasty patients in a highly cited study. They used a large nationwide administrative database maintained by Premier Perspective (Charlotte, North Carolina); the study data were gathered from 382,236 patients in approximately 400 acute care hospitals throughout the United States over 4 years.[11]

Other retrospective cohort studies comparing the occurrence of perioperative complications, such as surgical site infections (SSIs), cardiopulmonary morbidity, and mortality, have used the American College of Surgeons National Surgical Quality Improvement Program (NSQIP).[12–14] In an investigation by Liu and colleagues,[12] use of neuraxial anesthesia was associated with lower adjusted odds of both pneumonia and a composite outcome of any systemic infectious complication within 30 days of surgery when compared with general anesthesia (GA). NSQIP originally started within the Veterans Health Administration (VHA) system in the 1980s with a small sample of hospitals; this project, which included public reporting of outcomes data, eventually expanded to include all VHA surgical facilities and others outside the VHA system.[15] These data are entered by clinical staff, commonly nurses, at participating facilities and verified by chart review. In regional anesthesiology and acute pain medicine, multicenter prospective registries, such as the SOS Regional Anesthesia Hotline Service[16,17] and AURORA (Australia and New Zealand registry of Regional Anesthesia),[18,19] have been developed for outcomes research and have reported the occurrence rates of rare complications. For pediatric surgical patients specifically, a large prospectively collected multicenter database has been created and is called the Pediatric Regional Anesthesia Network.[20] The disadvantages to these data-driven studies include lack of randomization, which introduces potential bias; missing or incorrectly coded data; inability to draw conclusions regarding causation; and restrictions to access, such as information security issues and/or cost (eg, the Premier database). These retrospective cohort database studies, however, may offer large samples sizes and administrative data from actual real-world patients over a longer period of time and may identify important associations that influence clinical practice and generate hypotheses for future prospective studies. Pragmatic clinical trials are also used more frequently to address the effectiveness of certain interventions on a large scale. These studies, however, often require considerable time commitments, extensive organization, a high level of funding, and involvement of multiple institutions. An example of such a study is the ongoing trial to address the effect of Regional versus General Anesthesia for Promoting Independence after Hip Fracture (REGAIN).[21]

ANESTHESIA TYPE AND PERIOPERATIVE MORTALITY

Postoperative epidural analgesia was associated with significantly lower odds of death at 7 days (odds ratio [OR] 0.52; 95% CI, 0.38–0.73; $P = .0001$) and 30 days (OR, 0.74; 95% CI, 0.63–0.89; $P = .0005$) after surgery in a 5% random sample of Medicare beneficiaries from 1997 to 2001. This association was observed after adjusting for other risk factors across different surgeries.[22] Using similar methodology, the same research group queried a Medicare database to examine the effect of epidural analgesia on postoperative mortality and morbidity in total hip arthroplasty,[23] total knee arthroplasty (TKA),[24] colon resection,[25] and lung resection.[26] They concluded that epidural analgesia was not associated with decreases in postoperative mortality in total hip[23] and knee arthroplasty.[24] On the other hand, using epidural analgesia was associated with lower odds of death at 30 days after colectomy (OR 0.54; 95% CI, 0.42–0.70; $P<.0001$)[25] and lung resection (OR 0.53; 95% CI, 0.35–0.78; $P = .002$).[26]

Based on the study by Memtsoudis and colleagues,[11] overall 30-day mortality for lower extremity arthroplasty patients is lower for patients who receive neuraxial and combined neuraxial GA compared with GA alone. In most categories, the rates of occurrence of in-hospital complications are also lower for the neuraxial and combined neuraxial GA groups versus the GA-only group, and transfusion requirements are lowest for the neuraxial group compared with all other groups.[11] Wijeysundera and colleagues[27] analyzed population-based linked administrative databases from Ontario, Canada, to explore potential benefits for neuraxial anesthesia in intermediate to high-risk surgery. They reported a slightly lower rate (1.7% vs 2.0%) and relative risk (0.89 [95% CI, 0.81–0.98]; $P = .02$) of mortality compared with GA. These effects seemed more pronounced in orthopedic and thoracic surgery than in other surgical specialties. Using the same database, another study found no difference in 30-day all-cause mortality when adding spinal or epidural anesthesia to GA compared with GA alone in 21 different elective procedures (vascular, gastrointestinal, urologic, and thoracic).[28] Studies using NSQIP have reported no difference in 30-day mortality for carotid endarterectomy patients associated with anesthetic technique although regional anesthesia patients are more likely to have a shorter operative time and next-day discharge[14]; similarly, there is no difference in 30-day mortality for endovascular aortic aneurysm repair although GA patients are more likely to have longer length of stay and pulmonary complications.[29] In hip fracture surgery, regional anesthesia has been associated with lower adjusted mortality rates (OR 0.710; 95% CI, 0.541–0.932; $P = .014$) and lower rates of pulmonary complications (OR 0.752, 95% CI, 0.637–0.887; $P<.0001$) relative to GA.[30] Although these results were derived from analysis of the New York State hospital database, a second analysis[31] of the same database using instrument variable matching revealed similar mortality rates between the different anesthesia techniques.

Although some studies suggest that older and sicker patients, or those subjected to high surgical acuity, seem to benefit most from regional anesthesia,[30] recent evidence suggests that decreased odds for major complications and resource utilization after total joint arthroplasty may be achievable across all age groups, irrespective of comorbidity burden.[32]

INPATIENT FALLS AFTER JOINT ARTHROPLASTY

Regional anesthesia has been linked to inpatient falls in the setting of orthopedic surgery in general and specifically after joint arthroplasty.[33,34] Possible block-related mechanisms included weakness of the quadriceps muscle and loss of proprioception.[35] Memtsoudis and colleagues[36] analyzed Nationwide Inpatient Sample data files for patients undergoing joint arthroplasty between 1998 and 2007. They found that the incidence of falls was 0.85%, representing 2.1 falls per 1000 inpatient days. Major risk factors associated with falls included revision surgery, older age, male gender, and higher comorbidity index. Falls were associated with longer hospital length of stay. Additionally, these patients had higher mortality and more complications and were less likely to be discharged home versus other skilled nursing facility.[36] In a similar study[37] of patients undergoing joint arthroplasty included in the Premier database between 2006 and 2010, the incidence of falls was 1.6%. Patients who GA had a higher incidence of falls compared with neuraxial anesthesia patients. Peripheral nerve block (PNB) was not significantly associated with inpatient falls (OR 0.85 [95% CI, 0.71–1.03]).[37] This latest study,[38] and others, highlight the fact that quadriceps muscle weakness resulting from a PNB is not the only reason that patients fall. Multiple factors may contribute to falls, which calls attention to the importance of instituting a multidisciplinary fall prevention program at every institution that cares for joint replacement patients.[39,40]

ANESTHESIA TYPE AND INFECTION RATE

SSIs remain among the most common serious perioperative complications. Neuraxial anesthesia has been proposed as a preventive strategy against SSI. Plausible mechanisms include reducing nonspecific generalized inflammatory response to surgery.[41] Sympathectomy-induced vasodilation and subsequent improvement in tissue oxygenation may be a second mechanism. Additionally, use of epidural analgesia for postoperative pain management can result in a decrease in infection risk because severe pain can provoke an autonomic response which, in turn, can cause vasoconstriction and reduced peripheral perfusion. Although none of these potential mechanisms individually can explain the reduction in systemic infection, a combination of the 3 may substantially reduce infection risk.[41]

Chang and colleagues[42] used the Longitudinal Health Insurance Database of Taiwan to study the association between SSIs and the type of anesthesia after hip and knee arthroplasty. The odds of SSIs for patients receiving GA were 2.21-times higher (95% CI, 1.25–3.90; P = .007) than those who had the same procedure under epidural or spinal anesthesia, after adjusting for the patient age, gender, the year of surgery, comorbidities, surgeon age, and hospital teaching status.[42] Neuraxial anesthesia was also associated with lower odds of pneumonia and a composite outcome for systemic infection relative to GA in TKA patients.[12] These findings were the results of analysis of the NSQIP database between 2005 and 2010. This beneficial effect was corroborated in a meta-analysis of 13 studies between 1995 and 2015, including 362,029 patients.[43] On the other hand, Kopp and colleagues[44] conducted a retrospective case-control study and found no difference in the incidence of SSIs in patients undergoing total joint arthroplasty under general versus neuraxial anesthesia. It is clear that this is a promising area for study, and this relatively rare outcome lends itself to big data research methods.

PERIOPERATIVE ANALGESIA AND CANCER RECURRENCE

In a relatively small matched retrospective study, Exadaktylos and colleagues[45] have reported lower rates of recurrence and metastasis for breast cancer surgery patients who receive paravertebral analgesia versus conventional systemic opioids. Although the exact mechanism was not well understood at that time (regional anesthesia vs reduction in the use of anesthetic agents and opioids), clinical and basic science research in this area has grown rapidly and has demonstrated mixed results. A follow-up study involving 503 patients who underwent abdominal surgery for cancer and were previously enrolled in a large multicenter clinical trial[46] and a retrospective database study of 424 colorectal cancer patients who underwent laparoscopic resection[47] have not shown a difference in recurrence-free survival or mortality. A recent meta-analysis, including 14 prospective and retrospective studies involving cancer patients (colorectal, ovarian, breast, prostate, and hepatocellular) demonstrates a positive association between epidural analgesia and overall survival but no difference in recurrence-free survival compared with GA with opioid analgesia.[48]

ANALGESIC TECHNIQUE AND PERSISTENT POSTSURGICAL PAIN

Chronic pain may develop after many common operations, including breast surgery, hernia repair, thoracic surgery, and amputation, and is associated with severe acute pain in the postoperative period.[49] Although regional analgesic techniques are effective for acute pain management, currently available data are inconclusive with regard to their ability to prevent the development of persistent postsurgical pain (PPSP).[50–52] A Cochrane systematic review and meta-analysis reviewed published studies on this subject, and the results favor epidural analgesia for prevention of PPSP after thoracotomy and favor paravertebral block for prevention of PPSP after breast cancer surgery at 6 months.[53] The results of other studies do not agree, however. Another meta-analysis evaluating PPSP after breast surgery concludes that there is no difference in terms of PPSP at 6 and 12 months attributable to paravertebral block[51] whereas single-institution studies following-up patients after previously completed randomized clinical trials show less PPSP in patients who receive a single injection[50] or continuous[54] paravertebral block prior to breast surgery. For thoracotomy, both epidural analgesia and paravertebral block can provide effective acute pain management with fewer side effects associated with paravertebral block,[55] but only epidural has been associated with risk of developing PPSP.[52,53] Definitive conclusions, however, regarding the role of regional anesthesia techniques, especially peripheral nerve blocks, in the development of PPSP are difficult to make given the limitations of small sample sizes. This represents an opportunity to use larger databases to investigate this issue on a population level and perhaps use opioid prescription history as a surrogate outcome for PPSP.[56,57] To date, database studies of younger patients (<65 years old) have not shown a decrease is long-term opioid use in patients who received nerve blocks for TKA or shoulder surgery.[58,59] In addition, continuous regional anesthesia techniques and perineural infusion regimens tend to be limited to the first 2 days to 4 days postoperatively, which may not adequately match the pain trajectory of major surgeries.[60] This pain trajectory for knee replacement suggests that an infusion duration of 1 week to 2 weeks may be more appropriate and argues strongly against single-injection nerve block techniques.

ULTRASOUND FOR REGIONAL ANESTHESIA AND PATIENT SAFETY

In 2010, the American Society of Regional Anesthesia and Pain Medicine published a series of articles presenting the evidence basis for ultrasound in regional anesthesia.[61]

According to the article focused on patient safety, evidence at the time suggested that ultrasound may decrease the incidence of minor adverse events (eg, hemidiaphragmatic paresis from interscalene block or inadvertent vascular puncture), but serious complications, such as local anesthetic systemic toxicity (LAST) and nerve injury, did not occur at different rates based on the nerve localization technique.[62] Since then, a large prospective multicenter registry study has shown that the use of ultrasound in regional anesthesia does reduce the incidence of LAST compared with traditional techniques, presumably from decreasing inadvertent intravascular injection of local anesthetic.[19] Similar methodology may be applied to other rare complications associated with anesthetic interventions.

PERIOPERATIVE PAIN MEDICINE AND HEALTH CARE COSTS

Approximately 31% of costs related to inpatient perioperative care is attributable to the ward admission.[63] Anesthesiologists as perioperative physicians have an opportunity to influence the cost of surgical care by decreasing hospital length of stay through effective pain management and by developing coordinated multidisciplinary clinical pathways.[64,65] The biggest challenge in demonstrating whether or not regional anesthesia and analgesia improve outcomes is that these techniques rarely exist in isolation and are commonly part of clinical pathways that involve a multipronged approach to streamlining surgical care.[66,67] One way that anesthesiologists can promote the implementation of evidence-based protocols to improve patient outcomes is to take leadership roles in perioperative medicine, also known as the Perioperative Surgical Home concept.[68] Although regional anesthesiology and acute pain medicine play an important role in this model of care, the establishment of a coordinated system of care that puts the patient in the center and continually evolves is the true goal and more likely to demonstrate outcome benefits.[69–72]

UTILIZATION OF REGIONAL ANESTHESIA

Despite a lot of signals derived from database research about improved perioperative outcome with the use of regional anesthesia, and the potential to improve some long-term outcomes, regional anesthesia is still underutilized. In joint arthroplasty, use of neuraxial anesthesia hovers at approximately 25% in best estimates.[11] Use of PNBs after TKA is not any better. It is estimated that only 12.5% of patients undergoing TKA use PNBs.[73] This is the case around the country despite recommendation of regional techniques by the American Academy of Orthopaedic Surgeons[74] and adoption of regional anesthesia as an outcome metric for performance in TKA by the Joint Commission.[75]

In summary, regional anesthesia and analgesia hae been shown in multiple studies to improve select short-term outcomes for surgical patients. Few studies to date, however, have explored long-term outcome benefits and positive effect on rare adverse events primarily due to limited sample sizes. Access to big data through multicenter prospective registries, multinational clinical trials, or large administrative databases allows some exploration of these issues and may provide the necessary evidence to support more widespread integration of regional anesthesia and analgesia within perioperative care.

REFERENCES

1. Vetter TR, Goeddel LA, Boudreaux AM, et al. The perioperative surgical home: how can it make the case so everyone wins? BMC Anesthesiology 2013;13:6.

2. Vetter TR, Ivankova NV, Goeddel LA, et al. An analysis of methodologies that can be used to validate if a perioperative surgical home improves the patient-centeredness, evidence-based practice, quality, safety, and value of patient care. Anesthesiology 2013;119(6):1261–74.

3. Vetter TR, Pittet JF. The perioperative surgical home: a panacea or Pandora's box for the specialty of anesthesiology? Anesth Analg 2015;120(5):968–73.

4. Butterworth JF 4th, Green JA. The anesthesiologist-directed perioperative surgical home: a great idea that will succeed only if it is embraced by hospital administrators and surgeons. Anesth Analg 2014;118(5):896–7.

5. Prielipp RC, Morell RC, Coursin DB, et al. The future of anesthesiology: should the perioperative surgical home redefine us? Anesth Analg 2015;120(5):1142–8.

6. Aston G. Service-line management: a behind the scenes road to value. 2015. Available at: https://www.hhnmag.com/articles/3757-service-line-management-a-behind-the-scenes-road-to-value. Accessed March 10, 2017.

7. Knott A, Pathak S, McGrath JS, et al. Consensus views on implementation and measurement of enhanced recovery after surgery in England: Delphi study. BMJ open 2012;2(6) [pii:e001878].

8. Macario A, Weinger M, Truong P, et al. Which clinical anesthesia outcomes are both common and important to avoid? The perspective of a panel of expert anesthesiologists. Anesth Analg 1999;88(5):1085–91.

9. Institute of Medicine. To err is human: building a safer health system. 1999.

10. Ma Y, Mazumdar M, Memtsoudis SG. Beyond repeated-measures analysis of variance: advanced statistical methods for the analysis of longitudinal data in anesthesia research. Reg Anesth Pain Med 2012;37(1):99–105.

11. Memtsoudis SG, Sun X, Chiu YL, et al. Perioperative comparative effectiveness of anesthetic technique in orthopedic patients. Anesthesiology 2013;118(5):1046–58.

12. Liu J, Ma C, Elkassabany N, et al. Neuraxial anesthesia decreases postoperative systemic infection risk compared with general anesthesia in knee arthroplasty. Anesth Analg 2013;117(4):1010–6.

13. Radcliff TA, Henderson WG, Stoner TJ, et al. Patient risk factors, operative care, and outcomes among older community-dwelling male veterans with hip fracture. J Bone Joint Surg Am 2008;90(1):34–42.

14. Schechter MA, Shortell CK, Scarborough JE. Regional versus general anesthesia for carotid endarterectomy: the American College of Surgeons National Surgical Quality Improvement Program perspective. Surgery 2012;152(3):309–14.

15. Ingraham AM, Richards KE, Hall BL, et al. Quality improvement in surgery: the American College of Surgeons National Surgical Quality Improvement Program approach. Adv Surg 2010;44:251–67.

16. Auroy Y, Benhamou D, Bargues L, et al. Major complications of regional anesthesia in France: the SOS Regional Anesthesia Hotline Service. Anesthesiology 2002;97(5):1274–80.

17. Auroy Y, Narchi P, Messiah A, et al. Serious complications related to regional anesthesia: results of a prospective survey in France. Anesthesiology 1997; 87(3):479–86.

18. Barrington MJ, Watts SA, Gledhill SR, et al. Preliminary results of the Australasian Regional Anaesthesia Collaboration: a prospective audit of more than 7000 peripheral nerve and plexus blocks for neurologic and other complications. Reg Anesth Pain Med 2009;34(6):534–41.

19. Barrington MJ, Kluger R. Ultrasound guidance reduces the risk of local anesthetic systemic toxicity following peripheral nerve blockade. Reg Anesth Pain Med 2013;38(4):289–97.

20. Polaner DM, Taenzer AH, Walker BJ, et al. Pediatric Regional Anesthesia Network (PRAN): a multi-institutional study of the use and incidence of complications of pediatric regional anesthesia. Anesth Analg 2012;115(6):1353–64.

21. Neuman MD, Ellenberg SS, Sieber FE, et al. Regional versus General Anesthesia for Promoting Independence after Hip Fracture (REGAIN): protocol for a pragmatic, international multicentre trial. BMJ open 2016;6(11):e013473.

22. Wu CL, Hurley RW, Anderson GF, et al. Effect of postoperative epidural analgesia on morbidity and mortality following surgery in medicare patients. Reg Anesth Pain Med 2004;29(6):525–33 [discussion: 515–29].

23. Wu CL, Anderson GF, Herbert R, et al. Effect of postoperative epidural analgesia on morbidity and mortality after total hip replacement surgery in medicare patients. Reg Anesth Pain Med 2003;28(4):271–8.

24. Wu CL, Demeester JS, Herbert R, et al. Correlation of postoperative epidural analgesia with morbidity and mortality following total knee replacement in Medicare patients. Am J Orthop (Belle Mead NJ) 2008;37(10):524–7.

25. Wu CL, Rowlingson AJ, Herbert R, et al. Correlation of postoperative epidural analgesia on morbidity and mortality after colectomy in Medicare patients. J Clin Anesth 2006;18(8):594–9.

26. Wu CL, Sapirstein A, Herbert R, et al. Effect of postoperative epidural analgesia on morbidity and mortality after lung resection in Medicare patients. J Clin Anesth 2006;18(7):515–20.

27. Wijeysundera DN, Beattie WS, Austin PC, et al. Epidural anaesthesia and survival after intermediate-to-high risk non-cardiac surgery: a population-based cohort study. Lancet 2008;372(9638):562–9.

28. Nash DM, Mustafa RA, McArthur E, et al. Combined general and neuraxial anesthesia versus general anesthesia: a population-based cohort study. Can J Anaesth 2015;62(4):356–68.

29. Edwards MS, Andrews JS, Edwards AF, et al. Results of endovascular aortic aneurysm repair with general, regional, and local/monitored anesthesia care in the American College of Surgeons National Surgical Quality Improvement Program database. J Vasc Surg 2011;54(5):1273–82.

30. Neuman MD, Silber JH, Elkassabany NM, et al. Comparative effectiveness of regional versus general anesthesia for hip fracture surgery in adults. Anesthesiology 2012;117(1):72–92.

31. Neuman MD, Rosenbaum PR, Ludwig JM, et al. Anesthesia technique, mortality, and length of stay after hip fracture surgery. JAMA 2014;311(24):2508–17.

32. Memtsoudis SG, Rasul R, Suzuki S, et al. Does the impact of the type of anesthesia on outcomes differ by patient age and comorbidity burden? Reg Anesth Pain Med 2014;39(2):112–9.

33. Finn DM, Agarwal RR, Ilfeld BM, et al. Fall risk associated with continuous peripheral nerve blocks following knee and hip arthroplasty. Medsurg Nurs 2016;25(1):25–30, 49.

34. Ilfeld BM, Duke KB, Donohue MC. The association between lower extremity continuous peripheral nerve blocks and patient falls after knee and hip arthroplasty. Anesth Analg 2010;111(6):1552–4.

35. Ilfeld BM. Single-injection and continuous femoral nerve blocks are associated with different risks of falling. Anesthesiology 2014;121(3):668–9.

36. Memtsoudis SG, Dy CJ, Ma Y, et al. In-hospital patient falls after total joint arthroplasty: incidence, demographics, and risk factors in the United States. J Arthroplasty 2012;27(6):823–8.e1.

37. Memtsoudis SG, Danninger T, Rasul R, et al. Inpatient falls after total knee arthroplasty: the role of anesthesia type and peripheral nerve blocks. Anesthesiology 2014;120(3):551–63.

38. Elkassabany NM, Antosh S, Ahmed M, et al. The risk of falls after total knee arthroplasty with the use of a femoral nerve block versus an adductor canal block: a double-blinded randomized controlled study. Anesth Analg 2016;122(5): 1696–703.

39. Kim TE, Mariano ER. Developing a multidisciplinary fall reduction program for lower-extremity joint arthroplasty patients. Anesthesiol Clin 2014;32(4):853–64.

40. Johnson RL, Duncan CM, Ahn KS, et al. Fall-prevention strategies and patient characteristics that impact fall rates after total knee arthroplasty. Anesth Analg 2014;119(5):1113–8.

41. Sessler DI. Neuraxial anesthesia and surgical site infection. Anesthesiology 2010; 113(2):265–7.

42. Chang CC, Lin HC, Lin HW, et al. Anesthetic management and surgical site infections in total hip or knee replacement: a population-based study. Anesthesiology 2010;113(2):279–84.

43. Zorrilla-Vaca A, Grant MC, Mathur V, et al. The impact of neuraxial versus general anesthesia on the incidence of postoperative surgical site infections following knee or hip arthroplasty: a meta-analysis. Reg Anesth Pain Med 2016;41(5): 555–63.

44. Kopp SL, Berbari EF, Osmon DR, et al. The impact of anesthetic management on surgical site infections in patients undergoing total knee or total hip arthroplasty. Anesth Analg 2015;121(5):1215–21.

45. Exadaktylos AK, Buggy DJ, Moriarty DC, et al. Can anesthetic technique for primary breast cancer surgery affect recurrence or metastasis? Anesthesiology 2006;105(4):660–4.

46. Myles PS, Peyton P, Silbert B, et al. Perioperative epidural analgesia for major abdominal surgery for cancer and recurrence-free survival: randomised trial. BMJ 2011;342:d1491.

47. Day A, Smith R, Jourdan I, et al. Retrospective analysis of the effect of postoperative analgesia on survival in patients after laparoscopic resection of colorectal cancer. Br J Anaesth 2012;109(2):185–90.

48. Chen WK, Miao CH. The effect of anesthetic technique on survival in human cancers: a meta-analysis of retrospective and prospective studies. PloS One 2013; 8(2):e56540.

49. Kehlet H, Jensen TS, Woolf CJ. Persistent postsurgical pain: risk factors and prevention. Lancet 2006;367(9522):1618–25.

50. Kairaluoma PM, Bachmann MS, Rosenberg PH, et al. Preincisional paravertebral block reduces the prevalence of chronic pain after breast surgery. Anesth Analg 2006;103(3):703–8.

51. Schnabel A, Reichl SU, Kranke P, et al. Efficacy and safety of paravertebral blocks in breast surgery: a meta-analysis of randomized controlled trials. Br J Anaesth 2010;105(6):842–52.

52. Wildgaard K, Ravn J, Kehlet H. Chronic post-thoracotomy pain: a critical review of pathogenic mechanisms and strategies for prevention. Eur J Cardiothorac Surg 2009;36(1):170–80.

53. Andreae MH, Andreae DA. Regional anaesthesia to prevent chronic pain after surgery: a Cochrane systematic review and meta-analysis. Br J Anaesth 2013; 111(5):711–20.

54. Ilfeld BM, Madison SJ, Suresh PJ, et al. Persistent postmastectomy pain and pain-related physical and emotional functioning with and without a continuous paravertebral nerve block: a prospective 1-year follow-up assessment of a randomized, triple-masked, placebo-controlled study. Ann Surg Oncol 2015;22(6): 2017–25.

55. Davies RG, Myles PS, Graham JM. A comparison of the analgesic efficacy and side-effects of paravertebral vs epidural blockade for thoracotomy–a systematic review and meta-analysis of randomized trials. Br J Anaesth 2006;96(4):418–26.

56. Sun EC, Darnall BD, Baker LC, et al. Incidence of and risk factors for chronic opioid use among opioid-naive patients in the postoperative period. JAMA Intern Med 2016;176(9):1286–93.

57. Mudumbai SC, Oliva EM, Lewis ET, et al. Time-to-cessation of postoperative opioids: a population-level analysis of the veterans affairs health care system. Pain Med 2016;17(9):1732–43.

58. Sun EC, Bateman BT, Memtsoudis SG, et al. Lack of association between the use of nerve blockade and the risk of postoperative chronic opioid use among patients undergoing total knee arthroplasty: evidence from the marketscan database. Anesth Analg 2017;125(3):999–1007.

59. Mueller KG, Memtsoudis SG, Mariano ER, et al. Lack of association between the use of nerve blockade and the risk of persistent opioid use among patients undergoing shoulder arthroplasty: evidence from the marketscan database. Anesth Analg 2017;125(3):1014–20.

60. Lavand'homme PM, Grosu I, France MN, et al. Pain trajectories identify patients at risk of persistent pain after knee arthroplasty: an observational study. Clin Orthop Relat Res 2014;472(5):1409–15.

61. Neal JM, Brull R, Chan VW, et al. The ASRA evidence-based medicine assessment of ultrasound-guided regional anesthesia and pain medicine: executive summary. Reg Anesth Pain Med 2010;35(2 Suppl):S1–9.

62. Neal JM. Ultrasound-guided regional anesthesia and patient safety: an evidence-based analysis. Reg Anesth Pain Med 2010;35(2 Suppl):S59–67.

63. Macario A, Vitez TS, Dunn B, et al. Where are the costs in perioperative care? Analysis of hospital costs and charges for inpatient surgical care. Anesthesiology 1995;83(6):1138–44.

64. Ilfeld BM, Mariano ER, Williams BA, et al. Hospitalization costs of total knee arthroplasty with a continuous femoral nerve block provided only in the hospital versus on an ambulatory basis: a retrospective, case-control, cost-minimization analysis. Reg Anesth Pain Med 2007;32(1):46–54.

65. Jakobsen DH, Sonne E, Andreasen J, et al. Convalescence after colonic surgery with fast-track vs conventional care. Colorectal Dis 2006;8(8):683–7.

66. Macario A, Horne M, Goodman S, et al. The effect of a perioperative clinical pathway for knee replacement surgery on hospital costs. Anesth Analg 1998; 86(5):978–84.

67. Hebl JR, Kopp SL, Ali MH, et al. A comprehensive anesthesia protocol that emphasizes peripheral nerve blockade for total knee and total hip arthroplasty. J Bone Joint Surg Am 2005;87(Suppl 2):63–70.

68. Kain ZN, Vakharia S, Garson L, et al. The perioperative surgical home as a future perioperative practice model. Anesth Analg 2014;118(5):1126–30.

69. Walters TL, Howard SK, Kou A, et al. Design and implementation of a perioperative surgical home at a veterans affairs hospital. Semin Cardiothorac Vasc Anesth 2016;20(2):133–40.

70. Mudumbai SC, Walters TL, Howard SK, et al. The Perioperative Surgical Home model facilitates change implementation in anesthetic technique within a clinical pathway for total knee arthroplasty. Healthc (Amst) Dec 2016;4(4):334–9.

71. Walters TL, Mariano ER, Clark JD. Perioperative surgical home and the integral role of pain medicine. Pain Med 2015;16(9):1666–72.

72. Mariano ER, Walters TL, Kim TE, et al. Why the perioperative surgical home makes sense for veterans affairs health care. Anesth Analg 2015;120(5):1163–6.

73. Memtsoudis SG, Poeran J, Cozowicz C, et al. The impact of peripheral nerve blocks on perioperative outcome in hip and knee arthroplasty-a population-based study. Pain 2016;157(10):2341–9.

74. Treatment of osteoarthritis of the knee, evidence-based guideline. 2013; 2nd edition. Available at: https://www.aaos.org/research/guidelines/treatmentofosteo arthritisofthekneeguideline.pdf. Accessed March 15, 2018.

75. Disease-Specific Care,Advanced Certification Program. 2018. Available at: https://www.jointcommission.org/assets/1/6/THKRIP_Manual2018January_New. pdf. Accessed March 15, 2018.

Printed and bound by CPI Group (UK) Ltd, Croydon, CR0 4YY

08/05/2025

01864725-0003